Treatment planning in general dental practice

A problem-based approach

Dedication

To my wife Angela
for her loving companionship, patience and unending support

and to our children (young adults!), Gabrielle, Genevieve and Nicholas for putting up
with my major time commitments to dentistry and for turning out just fine.

Commissioning Editor: Michael Parkinson
Project Development Manager: Barbara Simmons
Project Manager: Frances Affleck
Designer: Judith Wright

Treatment planning in general dental practice

A problem-based approach

Crawford A. Bain BDS DDS MSc MBA

Senior Lecturer in Dental Primary Care
University of Glasgow Dental School
Glasgow

Series editor

F.J. Trevor Burke

Professor of Dental Primary Care
University of Birmingham School of Dentistry

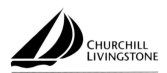

CHURCHILL
LIVINGSTONE

EDINBURGH   LONDON   NEW YORK   OXFORD   PHILADELPHIA   ST LOUIS   SYDNEY   TORONTO   2003

CHURCHILL LIVINGSTONE
An imprint of Elsevier Science Limited

First published 2003

ISBN 0443 071837

British Library Cataloguing in Publication Data
A catalogue record for this book is available from the British Library

Library of Congress Cataloging in Publication Data
A catalog record for this book is available from the Library of Congress

Notice
Medical knowledge is constantly changing. Standard safety precautions must be followed, but as new research and clinical experience broaden our knowledge, changes in treatment and drug therapy may become necessary or appropriate. Readers are advised to check the most current product information provided by the manufacturer of each drug to be administered to verify the recommended dose, the method and duration of administration, and contraindications. It is the responsibility of the practitioner, relying on experience and knowledge of the patient, to determine dosages and the best treatment for each individual patient. Neither the Publisher nor the authors assumes any liability for any injury and/or damage to persons or property arising from this publication.

The
Publisher's
policy is to use
**paper manufactured
from sustainable forests**

Printed in Spain

Preface

This book is offered as an aid to both the dental student entering the clinical years, trying to bring together the several apparently disparate clinical disciplines, and the new dentist setting out into a general practice setting that contains none of the artificial barriers to integrated care which exist in some dental schools. It is also hoped that this text will be of some assistance to the more experienced clinician, competent in many clinical procedures and taking on the more challenging dental problems that present today in an ageing dentate population anxious to preserve and enhance their dentition.

The term 'treatment planning' in the title of this text is used more to allow readers to recognise a familiar function in dentistry than because I feel it is the most appropriate descriptor of the concepts contained herein. 'Treatment' does not always denote 'care' for the patient. Too often the dental student's or dentist's interests are placed ahead of those of the patient when decisions on treatment are made and presented. Treatment can be provided but care is not necessarily given. This is discussed in some depth in Chapter 1 and is largely a result of requirements-driven curricula in some dental schools, and by financial considerations and irrationalities in many third party payment schemes.

It would perhaps be better to use the term 'care planning' since this is hopefully the objective of all well-meaning clinicians who set out to manage patients' problems. It is the author's hope that, in time, care planning may become the term of choice when future dentists sit down with future patients to develop appropriate care choices.

It is appropriate to acknowledge several mentors and colleagues who have had significant influence on the evolution of the ideas presented in this text. Dr Geoff Cowley, then of Glasgow University for first sparking my interest in periodontics; Dr Morton Amsterdam at Penn for teaching me to think and to plan total care for my patients with advanced problems; Dr Adri El Geneidy and Dr John Eisner, then of Dalhousie University, for their hard work in taking the problem-based approach to treatment planning from the theoretical to the practical level, and for developing the concept of priority-sequencing used in this book; Dr Barry Kenney and Dr Peter Moy for allowing me to spend a wonderful year with them at UCLA and for continuing to lead research in periodontics and dental implantology. Also thanks to Professor Trevor Burke for his encouragement in this venture and constant support during his time in Glasgow. Most of all, to over 25 years of classmates, undergraduate and postgraduate students in Glasgow, Dalhousie, Penn and UCLA, whose involvement in treatment-planning seminars and clinical care continues to provide stimulus and enjoyment.

Glasgow 2003

Contents

1 Principles of problem-based treatment planning

Most dentists graduate from dental school with a basic competence in several restorative, prosthetic and surgical procedures, as well as the ability to take a good history and carry out a clinical examination in the several clinical disciplines. The nature of dental education in most dental schools leads to a compartmentalised approach to the basic aspects of data gathering, with the various disciplines each having their own requirements for diagnostic information prior to initiating treatment. The patient's overall diagnostic information is often assembled in a haphazard fashion in various parts of the patient's record.

Dental students and new graduates often find it extremely difficult to take the diagnostic data assembled for a patient with complex problems and develop it into a logical treatment plan that will best address the patient's needs. This situation is not helped in many dental schools, where divisional or departmental requirements, which must be completed for graduation, often take precedence over the patient's best interests in the student's mind. This often leads to treatment that addresses the student's requirements rather than the patient's needs, and in extreme cases the treatment plan can be viewed as a 'menu', from which the student selects the various procedures required for graduation, rather than a logical sequence of therapy designed to manage the patient's dental problems.

While this piecemeal approach to the provision of dental care may well result in clinically satisfactory individual restorations or prostheses, the failure to address the patient's overall needs, and the neglect of underlying problems that are not a priority in the student's mind, can often lead to a progressive deterioration in the dental health of patients who are more susceptible to dental diseases. Figures 1.1–1.5 shows radiographs of a patient who faithfully attended a dental school at least once a year over a 22-year period, never missing an appointment and always responding to recall. Over this period, he received various dental procedures such as root canal fillings,

bridges and crowns, all technically satisfactory when viewed individually, but with no real effort to address the patient's overall needs. Although a gingivectomy was carried out at one point and it was twice noted that he needed 3-monthly professional cleanings for periodontal maintenance, this was never in fact provided, and when he was finally referred to the graduate periodontal clinic, several extractions were necessary. This, despite his faithful attendance, reasonable oral hygiene, and willingness to follow all advice given. *This patient received treatment—NOT CARE!*

Sadly, this is not an unusual case either in a dental school or in the general practice environment, where too often there is progressive deterioration despite the regular attendance of patients for recall. It is perhaps an inevitable outcome of a situation where the students' requirements are placed ahead of patients' needs. This form of dental education, known as the *student-focused curriculum*, was the norm in most dental schools until the 1980s and still persists in many

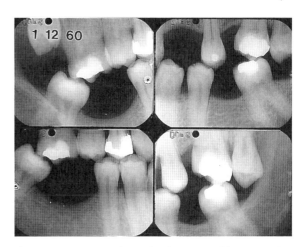

Figure 1.1 Bitewing radiographs of a 26-year-old patient on his first presentation at a dental school clinic in 1960 showing tooth loss without replacement, posterior bite collapse, unerupted and overerupted wisdom teeth. There is evidence of past caries management.

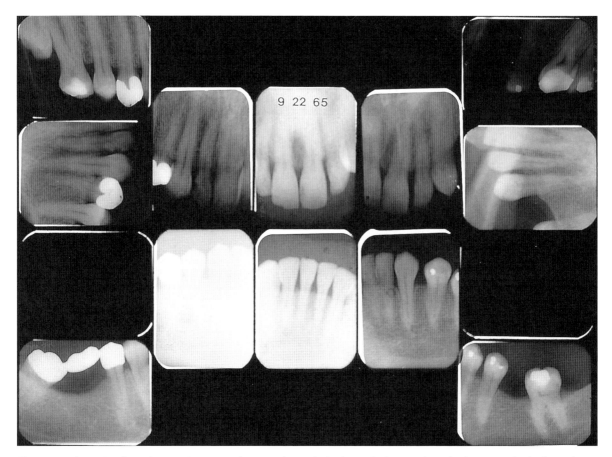

Figure 1.2 The patient from Figure 1.1 in 1965. He has now obtained a bridge on his lower right with a bizarre occlusal scheme (but good margins), as well as an upper premolar inlay.

today. We should not be too surprised when some within our profession, coming from such a dental school experience, continue to put themselves ahead of their patients, often using their patients, and the health service or other third party payment providers' in a less than ethical way. Although they must bear responsibility for their actions, dental educators who endorse the student-focused setting have certainly failed to provide a meaningful ethical role model for their students and, by default, endorse this 'me first' attitude. The teaching of bad practice by commission or by omission cannot be justified.

The patient in Figure 1.6 presented in 1982 with a failing reconstruction. This had originally been completed in Boston, Massachusetts in the 1960s. Periodontics had been carried out by the author of a standard text, as had endodontics. Restorative margins were perfect and yet all upper teeth had recently been extracted as a result of advanced periodontitis, and only three and a half lower teeth could be retained for a few more years. The patient had had virtually no maintenance for 15 years after the reconstruction. While regular maintenance had surely been proposed in the original treatment plan, the patient had not grasped the significance of this phase of treatment. It is fascinating to listen to dentists debate between chamfers and bevels for crown margins, between lateral and vertical condensation for endodontics, between gold and porcelain occlusal surfaces for crowns and bridges when the factor most likely to differentiate between success and failure is none of these, but the presence or absence of an adequate maintenance commitment from both patient and dentist. In this case, it is likely that the patient had viewed the treatment plan as a menu and chosen the parts he felt most necessary. He was lost to main-

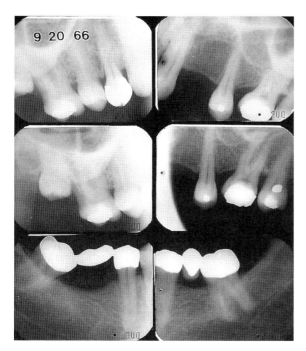

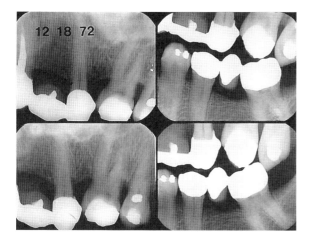

Figure 1.3 One year later (1966), the patient (from Figs 1.1 and 1.2) has another bridge on the lower left, with an equally unusual occlusal scheme.

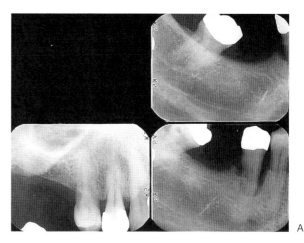

A

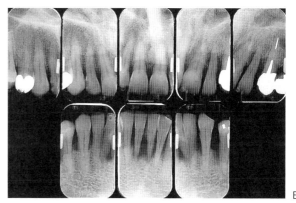

B

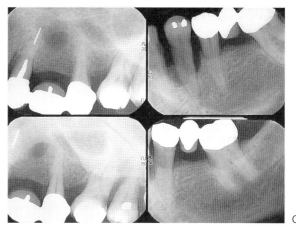

C

Figure 1.4 The patient shown in Figures 1.1–1.3 has another new bridge on the upper left in 1972. The upper left canine (previously a virgin tooth) has been root treated and has a large post. A plunger cusp has resulted from the relationship to the 1966 bridge and the patient, now aged 38, shows evidence of early bone loss. Soon after, 3-monthly periodontal maintenance was recommended but never provided. In 1976, a gingivectomy was performed on the upper molars: again after 3-monthly periodontal maintenance was advised and again not provided.

Figure 1.5 The patient now aged 48 has been referred to graduate periodontics. Molars on the upper right have been extracted due to advanced periodontitis; the lower right bridge has failed with significant bone loss on the anterior abutment and the upper left bridge is also failing due to an advanced endo/perio. All incisors have advanced bone loss and ultimately were extracted. So 22 years of 'care' has led to extensive partial dentures.

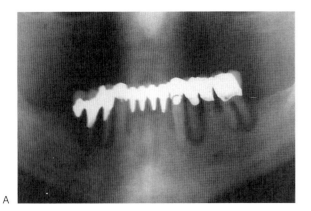

A

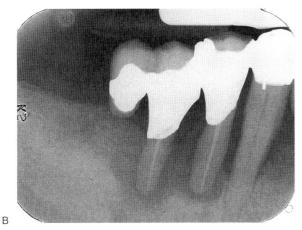

B

Figure 1.6 Failing reconstruction. (A) Panoramic radiograph (1982) of a 69-year-old lawyer with a upper and lower reconstructions originally completed by leading clinicians in periodontics, endodontics and bridgework. Restorative margins and root canal fillings were perfect and yet all upper teeth had recently been extracted because of advanced periodontitis, and only 3½ lower teeth could be retained for a few more years. The patient had failed to follow recall/maintenance recommendations. (B) A periapical view of this patient's lower right side. The high standard of endodontics and crown margins in no way compensates for the lack of periodontal maintenance.

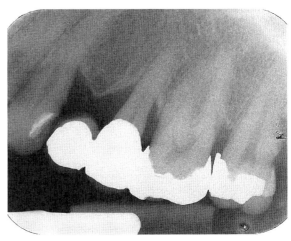

Figure 1.7 Advanced periodontitis on abutment teeth where a bridge was placed in the previous 6 months. Failure first to diagnose and treat underlying periodontal problems led to a successful malpractice claim.

tenance and ultimately became edentulous. Treatment was technically superb but lack of aftercare led to failure.

The patient in Figure 1.7 had recently had a bridge fitted to replace an upper left first premolar, by a dentist she had attended for 20 years. A periodontal abscess caused a referral (by another dentist) for periodontal treatment and 9 mm pockets with significant bone loss on abutment teeth were found. A subsequent request for old X-rays elicited only occasional bitewings over a 20-year period. No record of any periodontal diagnosis or treatment existed, nor of any oral hygiene instructions relating to the new bridgework. The dentist took the patient to collection for a small outstanding part of the bridge fee ($100); she subsequently countersued for malpractice and the case was settled for $19 000. Again the dentist selected those aspects of the patient's needs that he wished to treat and failed to treat or even diagnose her underlying periodontal problems. Treatment, not care, led to a need for major retreatment and considerable anguish for both patient and dentist.

The patient in Figure 1.8 had already undergone orthodontics twice, each time failing to comply fully with the retention phase of treatment. Now a dentist, she is about to go through orthodontics a third time; this time with more commitment to and appreciation of long-term retention. Again a failure to adhere to a part of the overall treatment plan led to relapse and a need for retreatment.

THE PROBLEM-BASED CURRICULUM

In the 1970s, at MacMaster University in Canada, the medical faculty developed an entirely new approach to teaching undergraduate medical students. By moving away from a lecture-based, student-focused curriculum towards group learning based on a series of carefully selected problems designed both to cover the core knowledge required and to develop the skills of the group in working together to find pertinent informa-

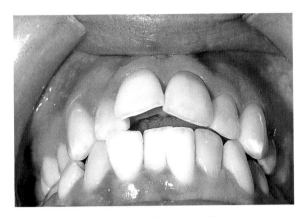

Figure 1.8 Orthodontic relapse has occurred in this patient, who has twice completed fixed orthodontics but has failed to follow retention recommendations. Again the *à la carte* approach to the treatment plan has led to failure and a need for retreatment.

tion, they developed what has now come to be known as a *problem-based curriculum*. So successful was this experiment that it has been widely imitated around the world and must now be considered as the norm in medical education. Several dental schools have also moved towards this type of curriculum.

The clinical part of the medical problem-based curriculum has resulted in the development of a patient's problem-oriented record, and the use of a problem list to organise the various signs and symptoms and to test results and aspects of medical and social history. This leads to a focal point from which a systematic approach to treatment is developed. The beauty of this approach is that it can be introduced to the entering first year medical or dental students and, after a brief introduction, used immediately at their own level of knowledge.

For example, a first year dental student, having had a basic review of what is normal, can examine a classmate's mouth and quickly develop a list of variations from the normal or of problems. These would be largely described in lay terms: an area of decalcification being described as a white spot, an anterior diastema being described as a space between front teeth, or gingivitis being described as red swollen gums. As the clinician gains knowledge and experience, technical terminology replaces the lay description, and insight into when active treatment is indicated, as against continued monitoring, will hopefully develop.

This problem-based approach to diagnostic data gathering is, however, so robust that it should not only serve the developing dental student well but also become an indispensable tool for the practising dentist, particularly in the examination and treatment planning of patients with complex problems. It is the purpose of this text to present a systematic approach to treatment planning for both students and clinicians in a general practice setting, which will serve them well in the management of the increasingly more complex situations that present in general dental practice.

Although this text has used the traditional title of 'Treatment Planning' a strong argument can be made for changing this descriptor to 'Care Planning' since, as the cases in this chapter illustrate, treatment does not necessarily imply care.

SUMMARY

This chapter has discussed the historical development of a problem-based approach to both teaching and treatment planning. It has illustrated the weakness of a 'student-focused approach' to clinical dental education, and its potential lasting effect on both the clinician's approach to patient management and the tacit endorsement of less than ethical approaches to care.

2 Data gathering

Although every dental student has been taught a systematic approach to examining the whole patient, the phrase 'open wide' has become synonymous with the *real* beginning of dental data gathering, to such an extent that it has become the title of a long-running humorous dental column. Indeed, some practice management gurus advocate so much delegation that the patient may well be seated in the dental chair, bib on, medical and even dental history filled out, and on occasion with radiographs taken and having had some dental hygiene treatment, before the dentist even arrives on the scene. We must again ask ourselves where the true 'patient focus' is in this approach? Is there too much truth in the old joke, oft repeated by patients, that the dentist only talks to the patient when his/her hands are already in the patient's mouth?

Historically, the fees for examination and treatment planning have never kept up with inflation, being seen as 'loss leaders' to bring the patient into the practice before the *real* dentistry begins. This misguided mantra, exemplified by the concept that real dentistry must involve the use a high-speed drill, and that we cannot charge as much for thinking as for doing something, has led to a focus on *doing the thing right* rather than *doing the right thing*. Lawyers, accountants and the like have little difficulty in charging healthy fees for thinking and advising rather than just *doing* something to their clients. They achieve incomes comparable with many dentists without resort to a high-speed drill and with considerable focus on taking a detailed history, and often a background literature review, before developing a plan for our detailed legal or financial care.

Figure 2.1 shows a radiograph of a fairly well-executed root canal filling on a premolar tooth, which will be very difficult to restore because of mesial drift. The patient's dentist had problems with retraction for a post and core impression and sent the patient for periodontal crown lengthening, in the vain hope that this would simplify crown construction. Since a large

filling was lost several months previously, no temporary restoration has been in place. The patient had not been advised of the mesial drift, which has reduced the space between the mesial of the molar and distal of the first premolar to less than the mesio–distal dimension of the second premolar. The distal of the second molar probed 9 mm with bleeding and a grade 2 furcation. There was recurrent caries distal to the first premolar. The dentist was so focused on trying to restore the second premolar, he had lost sight of the overall situation. No note had been made of the space loss by mesial drift and that the mesial-to-distal dimension of the tooth was greater than the distance between adjacent contact points. If this tooth is to be retained and subsequently crowned, some space regaining will be required. While the temptation is there to use a high-speed drill to reduce adjacent teeth, this is only a short term 'fix' since it would inevitably lead to poor embrasure spaces in a patient who already has periodontal problems.

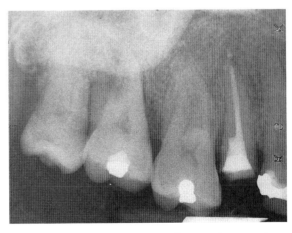

Figure 2.1 A radiograph of a fairly well-executed root canal filling on a premolar tooth. There is difficulty in restoring this tooth because of mesial drift. The patient was referred for crown lengthening.

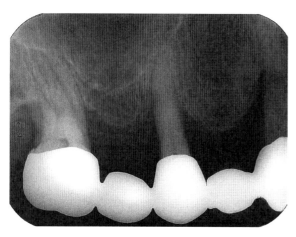

Figure 2.2 A five unit bridge placed in the previous 2 years on a patient with advanced periodontal disease who, although attending a dentist regularly, had never had sufficient management care.

Figure 2.2 shows a reasonably well-fitting bridge placed in the previous 2 years on a patient with advanced periodontal disease. The patient had attended a dentist every 6 months for the previous 8 years, had never had more than 15 minutes spent on scaling and had never been shown how to clean under the pontics. No mention of advanced periodontal disease had been made and bridges were proposed after the dentist had been on a crown and bridge course. While this bridge, and the root canal treatment in the patient illustrated in Figure 2.1, were technically well carried out as individual procedures, they were totally inappropriate procedures instituted without consideration and management of the overall situation. Again, the patient had received treatment, but not care.

With such a focus on procedures, it should not then be surprising that, when organised dentistry argues fees with third parties, there is generally pressure to advance the restorative procedures fees, usually at the expense of the diagnosis and treatment planning section in a fee guide.

MANAGING THE NEW PATIENT

When new patients arrive in a practice, they are entering unfamiliar surroundings and meeting new people. They are often anxious and may even be in pain. It is human nature to form fairly rapid opinions based on first impressions, and certainly the impression most dentists would hope to convey is that of a caring team

working in a calm, unhurried and clean environment. The patient would like to be made to feel the centre of attention and to experience individualised care.

Preliminary data

There is inevitably considerable preliminary data on the patient's demographics that must be assembled before the patient enters the treatment area. This includes full name, address, telephone numbers, date of birth and method of payment for services. It is also wise to gain information on occupation and next of kin with a contact phone number.

While some practices send out a 'patient welcome package' with a practice brochure and personal demographics form to fill out in advance, this may be perceived as 'too slick' or impersonal by older patients coming to the practice for the first time. There is also the risk that the patient may complete the form and forget to bring it with them, stimulating some resentment and delay when asked to complete it again. Perhaps a 'welcome package' is best limited to clear directions to the practice, advice on parking and brief curriculum vitae of staff members, outlining their qualifications, experience and areas of special interest.

It is wise to ask the new patient to come a few minutes early 'to do some paperwork'. Appropriately designed confidential forms can gather essential information both on patient demographics and on basic medical history while the patient is in the waiting area. In many practice locations, forms in more than one language may be needed, and by asking the patient to come early there should be no pressure to get them into the treatment area before forms are completed, and their initial few minutes in the practice will be spent occupied with the completion of the form rather than sitting with some level of anxiety until being taken through to meet the dentist.

The receptionist should know when a new patient is due and have sufficient preliminary information (name, age and gender) to recognise and make a friendly greeting, by name wherever possible.

> You must be Mr MacDonald? Our waiting room is just through here, make yourself comfortable and I'll just give you a little paper work to do. Would you like a tea, coffee, water or juice?

This is certainly better than 'And you are? Do you have an appointment today? What is it for?'

History taking

History taking involves documenting:

- chief complaint and wishes
- medical history
- dental history
- social history.

The key to effective history taking is to use well-selected, open questions, which allow the patient to supply necessary information without excessive digression and in a semi-structured manner that is easy to record. The classical medical sequence of history taking is well tested, but the dentist should modify his/her vocabulary to fit the individual in the chair.

Chief complaint and wishes

As the dentist is trying to establish the patient's main reason for being there, it is simplest then to ask: 'What is the main reason for you coming to see me today?' This will elicit a much more relevant information than closed questions such as 'Are you having any problems?' or 'Are you having pain?' Even if the patient answers yes to these questions, the dentist is a long way from finding out about the pain. Table 2.1 outlines appropriate and inappropriate opening lines to elicit the chief complaint.

With the gradual transition of modern dentistry from a purely health and management of disease service to include more quality of life and aesthetic issues, we have to elicit patient wishes as well as complaints. This focus on wants as well as needs should clearly establish what patients do not like about their mouths, while avoiding any impression of a hard sell. This can generally be determined by appropriate follow-up questions when the chief complaint does not identify these wants:

If there was one thing you could change about your teeth (mouth) what would it be?

How do you feel about the appearance of your teeth?

Are you happy with your smile?

Would you like to know more about what modern cosmetic dentistry can do for your mouth?

Medical history

While it is reasonable to gather initial health history data by a questionaire, it is imperative that the dentist goes over this with the patient to ensure that all questions were understood, and no confusion remains. Any ambiguous answers should be clarified, where possible, with the patient and, where necessary, with the patient's physician. The dentist should ensure that the patient understands why this information is necessary, when it may not have been elicited in such a thorough manner before. Older patients, in particular, are resistant to change and may need an explanation such as:

You know our parents and grandparents often lost their teeth when they were much younger than we are. It's a testament to dentistry that many people are keeping teeth much longer nowadays, but of course it means that we are now doing advanced treatment on our more senior patients, who may be on several new complex medications. That's why we have to be so thorough. What ever we do, we don't want to cause you any harm.

While many standard forms for medical history taking are available, and are generally comprehensive, the individual dentist should decide if any form he or she is considering contains all pertinent questions. If necessary, a form can be customised to include specific

Table 2.1 Establishing the reason for a dental visit

Appropriate (open) questions	Inappropriate (closed) questions
What is the main reason for you coming to see me today? Tell me how I can help you? Tell me what I can do for you? Is there anything special that you want me to do for you? Is there anything else that you particularly want me to investigate? Is there anything else that bothers you about your teeth? Are there any other improvements that you want in your mouth? Tell me more about . . .	Are you having any problems? Are you having pain? It's just a check up, is it?

questions not present on standard questionaires. It is, of course, important that the dentist knows why each question is asked, since the patient may well ask 'What has this got to do with my dental treatment?' This is particularly relevant with questions relating to sensitive and personal areas.

Examples of short and long medical history forms are to be found in the Appendix (p. 141).

The author recommends the use of the ASA (American Society of Anesthesiologists) physical status classification when considering the findings of the medical history and clinical data. Briefly, this classifies patients into five groups:

I   normal healthy patient

II   patient with mild-to-moderate systemic disease

III   patient with severe systemic disease that limits physical activity (is disabling) but is not incapacitating

IV   patient with severe systemic disease that limits activity (is incapacitating) and is a constant threat to life

V   a moribund (dying) patient not expected to survive 24 hours with or without an operation.

McCarthy (1972) in his excellent text expands in detail on special considerations necessary in each of these categories.

Dental history

The dental history can be an extremely useful part of history taking, since it often provides considerable insight into the patient's attitudes to dentistry. The dentist should try to obtain specific information where possible. Hence ask:

How often have you seen a dentist in the past?
Were there any long gaps between periods of treatment?

rather than

Have you been a regular attender in the past?

A patient's concept of what is *regular* may be very different from the dentist's. A patient who last saw a dentist 5 years previous for an extraction may still consider that this is their regular dentist, since they have seen no one else since, and plan to see the same dentist with their next problem!

Establishing the reasons for past visits will differentiate between the *regular recall attender* and

the *emergency only attender*. While it is reasonable to try to convert all patients into 'regular attenders', we must appreciate that individuals have their own priorities and concepts of how they wish to relate to dentistry. A successful general practice should provide several possible entry levels for patients, being inclusive rather than exclusive, while never losing sight of encouraging patients to upgrade the quality of their care.

Information on the nature and complexity of previous treatment will give some insight into the level of sophistication that the patient has been used to. Details of this can usually be elicited by a question such as: 'Have you ever had any complicated type of dental treatment in the past?'

We must remember that just because a patient has not experienced sophisticated treatment in the past does not mean that they do not wish advanced care. It may well be that they have not been offered anything beyond basic care. It does, however, indicate that more time may be needed to explain the options available, and the dentist must not expect immediate agreement to complex care from a patient only previously used to emergency or basic treatment.

It generally takes some time to establish a level of confidence and trust in a new patient, particularly when the type of dentistry that may be considered *ideal* for their problems is significantly different from their past experience. We may initially only 'sow seeds' while taking care of basic needs; provided active disease is stabilised, there is seldom a rush to carry out complex, reconstructive care. It often takes 2 or 3 years before a patient is comfortable enough with the dentist to progress to advanced care, and patients may choose to leave the practice if they feel they are being pushed too hard or too quickly. We should accept that patients will progress at their own rate, and that some may never go beyond accepting basic care.

Warning signs

Patient who has seen several dentists over the past few years. While this may be explained by frequent moves, it may also indicate a patient who holds dentists in fairly low regard ('They are all the same') or a patient who has unrealistic expectations or demands and cannot be satisfied by any of the previous practitioners. It may also be an indication of a patient who has bad debts with previous practitioners. It is wise to ask directly: 'You seem to have seen a lot of dentists over the years. What was it about your previous dentists that you found unsatisfactory?'

Patient who 'just knows' you can do something for them. Beware of the patient who is more confident in your ability to deliver a specific result than you are yourself. They are likely to have unrealistic expectations, and it is often the patient who 'just loves you' who can turn full circle and 'just hate you' if things are not exactly as they expect.

Patients with unrealistic time expectations. It is infinitely better to advise a patient that treatment is likely to take 8 months and then finish in 6, than to advise 6 months and take 8. Some patients attempt to push the dentist into a tight time frame, and generally there are too many variables beyond the direct control of the dentist to guarantee completion when you are being rushed. Either quality suffers or the treatment is not completed within the patient's time frame. Care should be taken before accepting a patient for any complex treatment where they are pushing to have it completed in significantly less time than would normally be required. Before committing to work in a constricted time frame, the dentist should weigh the potential benefits of attempting treatment under this type of time pressure against the potential ill-will created with staff and laboratories, the personal stress and the likely patient resentment if things do not go smoothly.

Patient who cannot remember the names of past dentists. This often indicates someone for whom dentistry is of little importance. It is likely that they will only proceed slowly to more advanced care and will often present only when a problem develops. It may also indicate a patient who does not want you to contact a former dentist.

Value of previous records The dentist examines a patient at one point in time. In essence, the examination data are a still photograph of a moving object. We can see where things are at present but not how fast they are going. Old records, particularly radiographs and study casts, can provide a valuable insight on the rate of progression of disease. Change, or lack of change, in bone levels, enamel caries and post-endodontic apical areas on radiographs, and wear facets, recession, diastemas, tooth tipping or overeruption on models, can assist us in differentiating between a stable and deteriorating situation. This, in turn, will allow us to decide if a problem is active, requiring treatment, or inactive requiring only monitoring. It will also allow

us to provide a more accurate assessment of prognosis to the patient. Obviously, a patient presenting with 50% bone loss today, who had 40% bone loss 10 years ago, has a better prognosis than a patient who only had 10% bone loss 10 years ago. Past records can turn the still picture into a moving one, giving objective information on change over time.

Patient A was referred in 1985 aged 42 years for restorative care. She clearly had advanced periodontitis with loss of a stable posterior occlusion, reduced vertical dimension and anterior flaring (Fig. 2.3A, B). Radiographs (Fig. 2.3C) showed between 30 and 100% bone loss on the remaining teeth. How can the clinician decide on the relative risk of undertaking complex perio-prosthetic treatment on such a patient. Advanced bone loss at such a relatively young age, combined with several missing posterior teeth, suggests an aggressive form of periodontitis. Current radiographs are like a still picture of a moving car. They show you the situation at one point in time but not the speed of change. Assembling old radiographs where these are available allows the clinician to develop a moving picture of the rate of progression of disease. Such films were obtained from previous dentists covering the period from 1965 to 1976 (Figs 2.4 and 2.5). These showed early bone loss already present in 1965. They also showed molar tooth loss was likely a consequence of caries not periodontal disease and that the present bone loss had developed over a 20-year period, not rapidly in recent years. This, combined with no history of any active periodontal treatment in the past, led the author to conclude that a major reconstruction was a reasonable risk in this patient. Treatment involved extensive periodontal root planning and surgery, extractions, endodontics and full upper and lower reconstructions to a shortened dental arch, followed by rigid maintenance. This was completed in 1985 and was stable, having only needed minor porcelain repairs, when the patient was last seen in 1995.

Contrast this with the patient illustrated in Figures 2.8–2.13. This patient presented in 2001 with advanced bone loss at age 61. One might reasonably assume that this had been slowly progressive over adult life. When, however, radiographs from 1995 were obtained (Figs 2.8–2.13, parts A), it became immediately apparent that bone loss and indeed tooth loss were rapid over the previous 6 years. History taking revealed a former heavy smoker (30+ pack-years; see below in Social history) who had adult-onset diabetes and admitted to a clenching and grinding habit. The overall prognosis

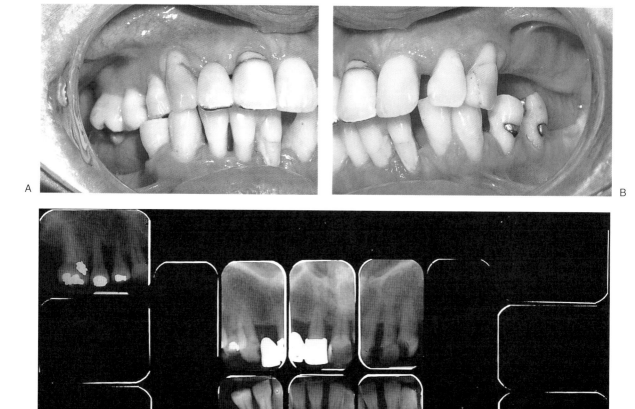

Figure 2.3 Patient A: an example of previous records assisting treatment decisions. (A,B) A 42-year-old patient with advanced periodontitis, loss of a stable posterior occlusion, reduced vertical dimension and anterior flaring. (C) Radiographs show between 30 and 100% bone loss on the remaining teeth.

was correspondingly poorer. It became necessary to treatment plan beyond the loss of most if not all teeth.

Seeking old records allows a dentist to communicate with former dentists, which will often clarify any confusion on past history. Patients are often vague on why teeth were extracted, on the specific details and frequency of past treatment. Medico-legal conventions (rules) vary from country to country on the ownership of patient records. It is generally wise to have a patient

sign a simple release of records such as the one shown in the Appendix (p. 141) and forward this with a covering letter to the former dentist(s). More details are discussed in Chapter 9.

Social history

While no one enjoys an unwarranted invasion of their privacy, there are certain aspects of the patient's social history that have direct relevance to their overall dental care.

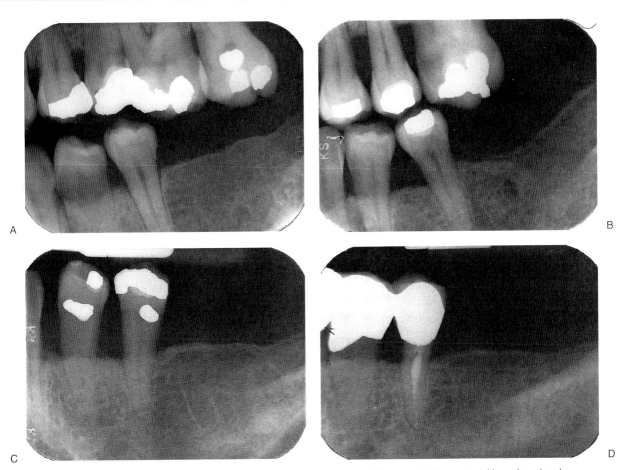

Figure 2.4 Patient A radiographic history. (A–C) The patient's lower left from 1965 until 1985 shows mesial bone loss already evident on the second premolar at age 23 (in 1965). Molars were already missing in 1965, almost certainly from caries *not* periodontal disease. (D) In 1988 after treatment.

Smoking Smoking habits are important to determine. This should be recorded as both daily consumption and number of years smoking, which is used to establish pack-years of use (daily consumption × number of years smoking).

A patient with 20 pack-years of smoking is not only at significantly increased risk of oral cancers but is also four to six times more likely to loose teeth through periodontal diseases. Dental implants are at least three times more likely to fail in smokers than non-smokers.

A patient who answer 'No' to being a smoker should be asked if they ever smoked, and if so how much and for how long. While there is ample evidence of the association between smoking and periodontal break-down, there is much less evidence that stopping smoking reduces or reverses the risk. Consequently,

information on past smoking history is important in developing a full picture of the factors contributing to the patient's present condition.

Alcohol Alcohol consumption is a precipitating factor for oral cancer in smokers; excessive alcohol consumption, particularly in binge drinking or associated with high sugar or citrus mixes, is also likely to be associated with erosive dental problems. Alcoholics are likely to be less-reliable attenders. The dentist should convert the information into units of alcohol per day or per week. It is almost useless to record a generalisation such as 'social drinker', which can mean many different things to different people. It is often best to ask 'Could you give me an idea of how much alcohol you consume in the course of a week?

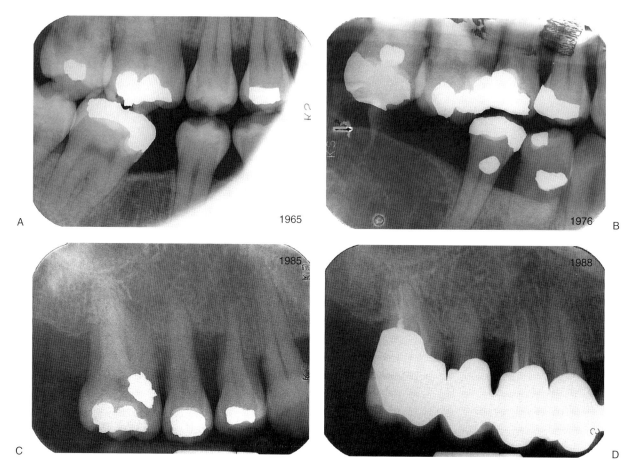

Figure 2.5 Patient A radiographic history. (A–C) The patient's right side between 1965 and 1985 again showed bone loss in 1965, and subgingival calculus. Caries likely caused the loss of lower right molars between 1965 and 1976. (D) In 1988, after treatment.

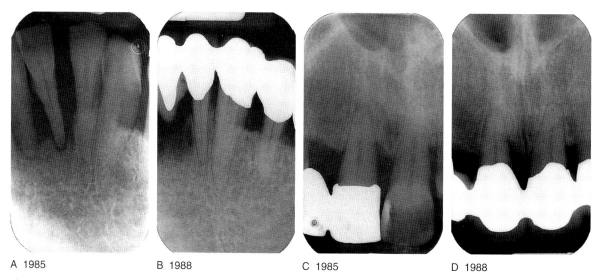

Figure 2.6 Patient A: radiographs of the incisors before (A,C) and after (B,D) comprehensive care. After reconstructive care, the bone levels around retained incisors have stabilised and some regeneration is evident.

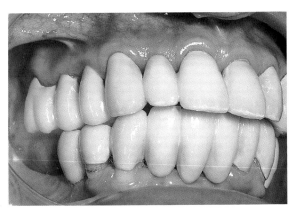
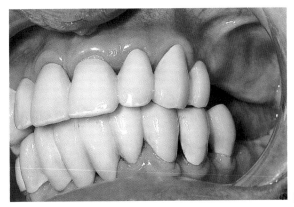

A

B

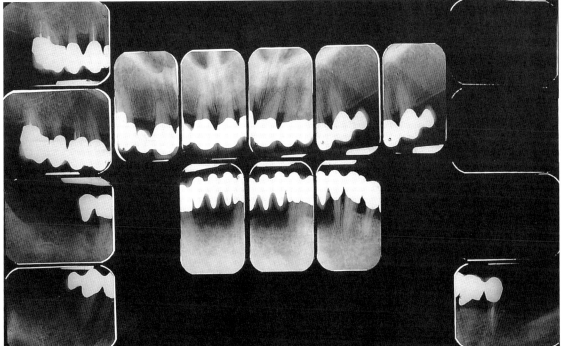

C

Figure 2.7 Patient A: completion of treatment 1 year later.

What type of things do you enjoy drinking?' rather than 'How many units of alcohol do you have each day?' or 'Are you a social drinker?'

Occupation Occupation will not only give an idea of the patient's educational and intelligence level but will also give an indication of potential levels of stress and, on occasion, availability for treatment. This information may well influence how the dentist approaches the explanation of any findings.

Personal situation Family situation and marital status will both identify potential additional patients, if other family members do not already attend your practice, and may also indicate potential stress in the recently divorced, widowed or the older single patient.

When any surgical or long and potentially arduous restorative procedure is planned, it is important to havea record of a contact number for a spouse, partner or other responsible adult, who can be contacted if the

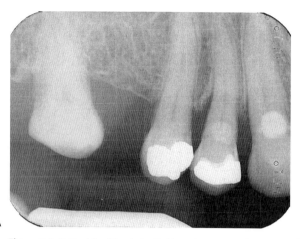
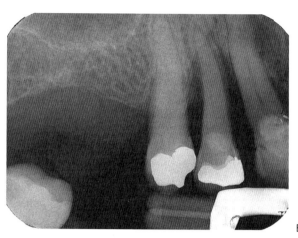

A

B

Figure 2.8 Patient B with substantial bone loss over a 6-year period. The upper right posterior region showing loss of second molar and massive increase in bone loss on first premolar from 1995 (A) to 2001 (B).

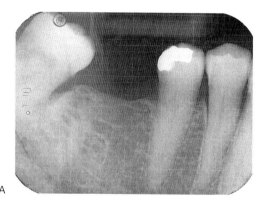
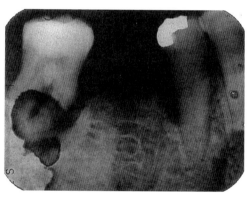

A

B

Figure 2.9 The lower right posterior region in Patient B again shows rapid bone loss over 6 years (A, 1995; B, 2001). Note the heavy calculus mesial to the second molar.

patient requires an escort home. Clearly with any type of sedation, a responsible adult escort in mandatory.

Stress history It is, on occasion, appropriate to ask directly about stress. This may relate to a chief complaint of facial pain, apthous ulcers, clicking joints, clenching and grinding or wear facets, and repeated tooth or filling fractures—as well as more rapid periodontal breakdown. It is usually effective to ask 'Have you had any particular increase in stress in the past few years?' This allows a general answer but does not force the patient to go into details unless they wish to. A follow up of 'Do you anticipate that the stress will reduce in the near future?' will generally furnish all the diagnostic information needed, while allowing the patient to go into details only if they feel comfortable to do so. Again it is important that the patient understands why this information is important, so that they do not feel that you are prying unnecessarily into private areas. Clearly the stress related to one specific event, such as a university final examination, while significant will generally be short in duration, while chronic situations such as a troubled marriage, handicapped child or business problems are likely to be ongoing in the longer term and will need continued consideration.

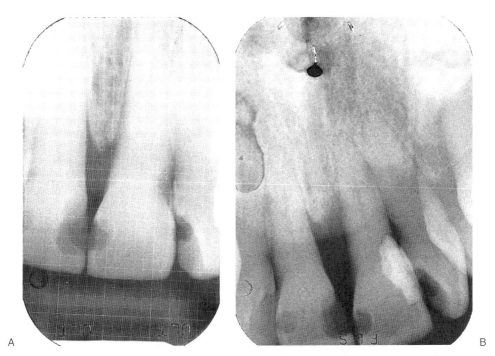

A   B

Figure 2.10 Again bone loss on upper incisors in Patient B has progressed from 30% at age 55 (A) to 70% at age 61 (B). This is clearly a form of late-onset rapid progression.

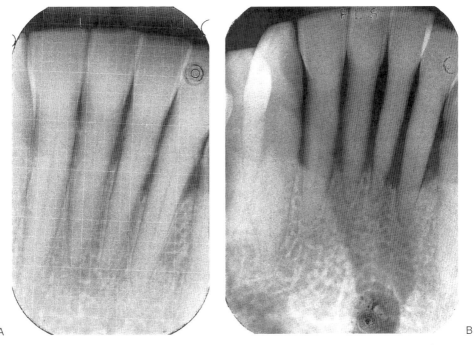

A   B

Figure 2.11 Patient B's lower incisors show progression from 50% (A) to 90% (B) bone loss over the same 6-year period.

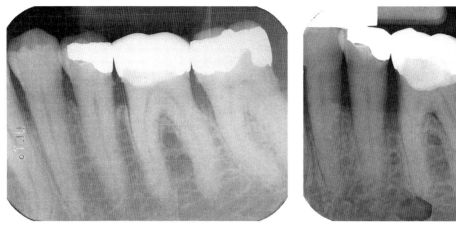

A   B

Figure 2.12 The lower right posterior region again shows a progression in bone loss from that in 1995 (A), leading to furcation involvement on the second molar which has also started to overerupt (B).

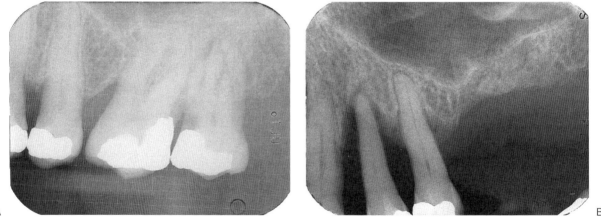

A   B

Figure 2.13 The upper left posterior region in Patient B shows loss of both molars and massive increase in bone loss on the premolars between 1995 (A) and 2001 (B). Note the widened periodontal ligament spaces due to secondary occlusal trauma and the increased loading resulting from loss of molars.

CLINICAL EXAMINATION

The clinical examination includes:

- extraoral aspects
- intraoral structures
- screening to assess needs for specialised examinations and tests.

Since much of the teaching in dental schools is carried out by specialists, it is not uncommon for the new graduate to be well trained in very detailed specialist examinations in individual disciplines, usually carried out on patients who have been preselected or referred because of specific problems in that discipline. When all of these various detailed examinations are combined, the total time involved is totally impractical for a general dental examination. The weakness of such teaching is that the new graduate often enters practice with little insight into what constitutes a comprehensive general examination, and when a more detailed specialist examination is indicated. It is the purpose of this text to detail what is involved in a comprehensive general dental examination, including necessary screening in various specialist areas. The reader is referred to various specialist texts for details of a specialist examination where one is indicated.

General dental examination

Preliminary extraoral observations

The extraoral examination starts as the patient enters the treatment area, when the clinician should greet the patient, while observing their gait and demeanor.

- Is the patient breathless or sweating; does the patient appear old for their age?
- Is their complexion healthy (well oxygenated) or do they display pallor, cyanosis, yellowness or excessive redness?
- Is their handshake firm and dry, or limp, cold and clammy?
- Is there a general symmetry to their body or an obvious asymmetry?
- Do they maintain eye contact or avoid it?
- Do they speak clearly or not?
- Are they clean and neat or otherwise?

All of these observations may have a bearing on overall treatment planning and how the patient is best approached when findings and recommendations are presented.

Extraoral head and neck examination

Symmetry There is an expectation of a general bilateral symmetry when assessing the patient from the front. Particular attention should be paid to the relationship of nose, eyes and chin. These should be considered with the patient at rest, with teeth in the intercuspal position and as the patient moves to full opening of the jaw. Where any deviation occurs, this should be correlated to any noises elicited from the temporomandibular joints. Where a clear asymmetry is identified, a more detailed history of head and neck trauma should be elicited, and consideration should be given to the need for additional radiographs to differentiate skeletal asymmetry from soft tissue asymmetry (Fig. 2.14). Maximum opening should be measured. Generally an opening of three finger widths is considered normal but this obviously depends on initial overbite and finger width. It is better to use a Boley gauge (Fig. 2.14F). Average opening between incisors is 40–45 mm in females and 45–50 mm in males. By assessing strained and unstrained maximum openings and noting the location of any discomfort, the operator can often identify the source of an obstruction to opening. Since the rotation phase of opening generally occupies the first 25–30 mm of opening, a patient who cannot open beyond this point may well have an anterior displaced disc without reduction and is then not likely to have a click on the affected side.

Muscles Although dental students become familiar with the muscles of mastication during the study of anatomy, this knowledge in too often forgotten by the time they embark on clinical dentistry. It is both simple and informative to make a brief assessment of masseters (Fig. 2.15A), vertical and horizontal fibres of temporalis (Fig. 2.15B,C) and sternomastoid muscles (Fig. 2.15D), the trapezius (Fig. 2.15E) and medial pterygoid (Fig. 2.15F). The clinician should assess these with the patient both at rest and clenching. Intraoral palpation on the insertion of temporalis at the chorenoid process is possible (Fig. 2.16), and the consolidation of muscle fibres at this point is often an area of tenderness to palpation. Note should be made of both hypertonicity and tenderness. Again, positive findings should be related to other extraoral and intraoral findings.

Glands Palpation of the supraclavicular lymph nodes should be part of a basic cancer screening within the general dental examination of all new and recall patients. More specific examination of glands is appropriate when the patient presents with a possible infection. The reader is referred to several excellent texts on oral medicine for details of this examination.

Temporomandibular joints Palpation of the temporomandibular joint (TMJ) both laterally (Fig. 2.17A) and intra-auricularly (Fig. 2.17B) should be carried out both with the patient closed in the intercuspal position and during opening, closing and lateral jaw movements. Both tenderness and the timing of any joint noises should be noted and related with deviation on opening as discussed above.

Intraoral examination

A systematic series of circuits of the mouth is recommended. These should consist of:

- soft tissues
- teeth
- periodontium.

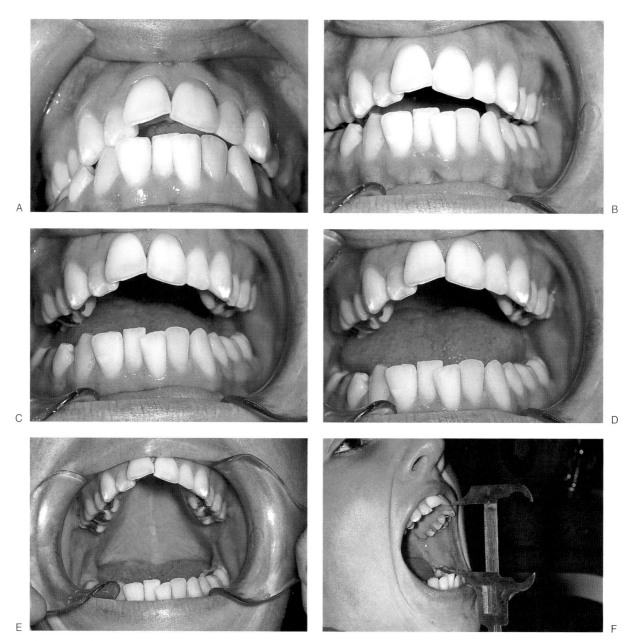

Figure 2.14 The symmetry of opening of the jaw. (A) The patient is in intercuspal position. Note that the upper midline is above the mesial of the lower left central incisor. (B) The patient opens a few millimetres to rest position. Already there is a slight deviation to the right. (C) With increased opening, there is a progressive deviation to the right until there is a click in the right temporomandibular joint. (D) As opening continues after the right joint click, the mandible starts to deviate back to the left. (E) At maximum opening the incisors are in the same alignment as at rest position. (F) The patient's maximum opening is measured. Generally the operator would measure unstrained and strained maximum openings and note presence and location of any discomfort associated with the strained position.

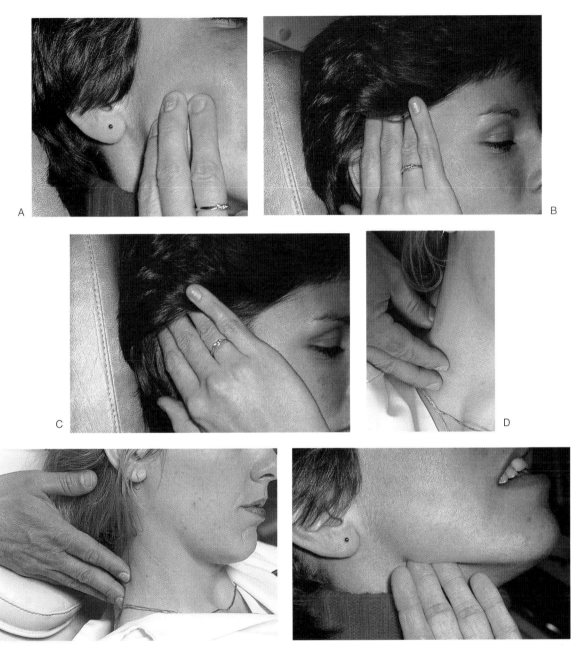

Figure 2.15 External examination of the facial muscles. (A) By first asking the patient to clench, the dentist can clearly identify the anterior border of the masseter. This should be palpated with two or three fingers and assessed for both tenderness and hypertonicity. (B) Again with the patient clenching, the vertical fibres of the temporalis muscle are assessed. (C) Palpation of the horizontal fibres of the temporalis muscle. (D) By asking the patient to turn her head to the opposite side, the sternocleidomastoid muscle becomes prominent. It should be palpated from clavicle to mastoid process. (E) From the supine position, the patient should lift her head from the headrest and let it drop back with the operator's hands taking the weight. The operator can then palpate the outer aspects of the trapezius muscle from shoulders to occipital bone. (F) By bringing the fingers from below the inner aspect of the lower border of the mandible and then pressing laterally, the dentist can palpate the superficial fibres of the medial pterygoid.

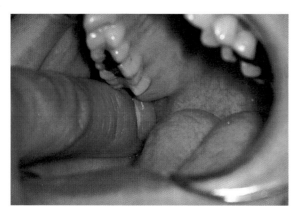

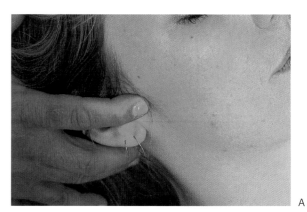

Figure 2.16 An intraoral assessment of the insertion of the temporalis muscle. By running a finger up the anterior border of the ascending ramus, the dentist will come to the insertion of the temporalis. This area often shows tenderness in patients with parafunctional habits.

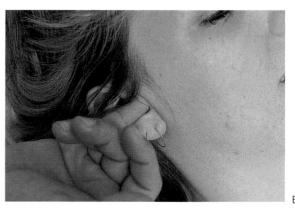

A

B

Soft tissues The soft tissues to be examined are:

- lips
- cheeks
- dorsum and underside of the tongue
- hard and soft palate
- throat.

A visual inspection should be carried out. The clinician must be familiar with normal appearance of these areas and alert to note all variations from the norm. Any red or white areas, as well as any raised or erosive lesions, should be palpated for discomfort and correlated with other aspects of the patient's history such as recent trauma, smoking or drinking habits.

Teeth An examination of the teeth should look for:

- missing teeth
- drifting
- tipping
- overeruption
- spacing
- existing restorations
- defective restorations
- caries
- excessive non-carious tooth structure loss (occlusal wear, abrasion, erosion or trauma).

Figure 2.17 Assessment of the temporomandibular joint. (A) The dentist should have the patient open and close until the outer aspect of the condyle is identified. The patient is then asked to open, close and move the mandible to left and right from a mid-open position. Tenderness, joint noises and limitations in movement should be noted. (B) The dentist places the small fingers in each external auditory meatus. Pressure is applied forward towards the retrodiscal area, and the patient again asked to open, close and move the mandible to left and right from a mid-open position. Tenderness, joint noises and limitations in movement should again be noted. Retrodiscitis is often associated with anterior disc displacement and associated joint noises.

Before a detailed examination for pathology is carried out, a baseline record of the number and position of teeth is needed. A clear record of all missing teeth should be made. Any drifting, tipping, overeruption or spacing should be noted. Existing restorations should be charted; defective restorations and active caries noted. The presence of non-carious tooth structure loss appears to be an increasing phenomenon presenting significant challenges both in diagnosis and management.

Periodontium An examination of the periodontium includes:

- periodontal probing depths
- assessment of mobilities
- assessment of recession over 1 mm
- bleeding on probing
- fremitus (functional contact mobilities).

For many years, the periodontal aspect of a general dental examination has been the poor cousin of caries examination and other aspects of charting. The large number of probing sites per tooth, often combined with an absence of appropriate periodontal probes in many practices, have led to its relative neglect. The advent of well-tested screening tools, the increased retention of many teeth to middle years and beyond, as well as the increase in litigation for failure to diagnose periodontal problems, has led to an increase in periodontal awareness on the part of many within the profession.

The development of the Community Periodontal Index of Treatment Needs (CPITN) as an epidemiologic screening tool (Ainamo et al., 1982), and its adoption under the guise of the Basic Periodontal Examination (PBE) in Britain and as Periodontal Screening and Recording (PSR) in North America has greatly facilitated periodontal screening in general practice. By using the World Health Organization (WHO) periodontal probe with lines at 3.5 and 5.5 mm, as well as a 1 mm rounded end, scoring runs from 0 to 4 (Table 2.2). The operator records only the highest score in each quadrant. Hence in a mouth of 32 teeth, only six numbers may be recorded rather than the 192 probings in a comprehensive examination.

Fundamental to the use of the BPE is the use of follow-up criteria, triggered by certain scores. A single score of 3 mandates full probings within that sextant while if two sextants have scores of 3, or one sextant has a score of 4, then full mouth probings as well as other aspects of periodontal examination are mandatory. It is fundamental to proper periodontal care in general practice that the dentist follows up positive BPE findings with the indicated action. This necessitates use of a periodontal examining probe such as a Williams or Michigan probe (Fig. 2.18A). The CPITN probe is purely for screening, not for full periodontal examination and follow-up (Fig. 2.18B).

Also part of the basic periodontal screening should be the recording of increased mobilities, recession

Table 2.2 The WHO Community Periodontal Index of Treatment Needs (CPITN)

Score	Periodontal status	Treatment needs
0	Healthy periodontium	No treatment needed
1	Bleeding observed	Oral hygiene instruction
2	Calculus felt; probe <3.5 mm; mobility[a] II (= I+)	Professional scaling
3	Pocket probes 4 or 5 mm; mobility[a] II (= I+)	Professional scaling
4	Pocket ≥ 6 mm; mobility[a] III (= I+/II+)	Complex treatment[b]

[a]Mobility using the Miller scale; see text.
[b]May include scaling and root planning under local anaesthetic and/or surgical exposure for access.

over 1 mm and bleeding on probing. While the last is often considered an indicator of active disease, this has recently been questioned, since smokers, who are a high-risk group for destructive periodontal disease, will tend to have less gingival bleeding than non-smokers with similar levels of breakdown, because of their compromised periodontal blood supply.

The Miller classification of mobility is still the most widely accepted. The operator uses two mirror handles or equivalent blunt instruments to rock the teeth in a bucco-lingual direction. The grades recorded are:

I   mobility of up to 1 mm

II   mobility between 1 and 2 mm

III mobility > 2 mm and/or compressible.

To this, many clinicians add a + or half unit to provide additional refinement to the scale.

A record of **fremitus** when the patient first taps in the intercuspal position and then in lateral and protrusive excursions is a useful indicator of occluso-traumatic problems and is particularly valuable when mobilities appear excessive in relation to radiographic bone levels. While access for measurement is limited compared with the open mouth recording of mobility, and hence only generally allows easy access to the upper anterior and premolar teeth, it does present a more accurate picture of what is actually happening during functional and parafunctional movements than does mobility. An unopposed molar with no

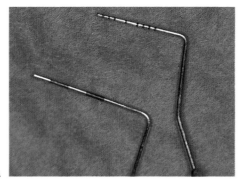

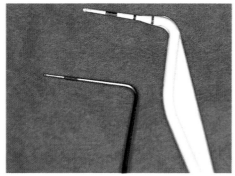

Figure 2.18 Basic periodontal examination. (A) The Williams probe (top) and Michigan probe (bottom) are designed for use in a comprehensive periodontal examination. These allow specific millimetre measurements for six sites per tooth. (B) The CPITN probe is available in metal or plastic versions. it is specifically designed for screening *not* for comprehensive periodontal examination. Its rounded tip is designed to detect calculus while avoiding unnecessary tissue trauma. The black strip runs from 3.5 to 5.5 mm and demarcates the scores of 1 and 2 (both below 3.5 mm) from 3 (3.5–5.5 mm) and 4 (above 5.5 mm).

contact with any other adjacent or opposing tooth may well have a mobility of 2 recorded on clinical examination; however, since this tooth is likely never rocked side to side, except during dental examination, this measure of mobility has little clinical relevance, unless increased loading via a partial denture or bridge is planned.

Fremitus, by comparison, records movements during function and parafunction which actually happens, usually many times per day. Although there has been extensive debate for many years as to the role of occlusal traumatism in periodontal breakdown, it is now generally accepted that, while not initiating loss of periodontal attachment, occlusal trauma can accelerate periodontal breakdown. Hence a finding of fremitus in the presence of loss of periodontal

attachment may well indicate an occluso-traumatic factor to be considered in treatment planning.

Fremitus is measured by placing the finger tips to the buccal of the upper teeth and then asking the patient to first tap in the intercuspal position, and then go through protrusive and lateral movements with the teeth in contact. If mobility is felt, then the operator removes his fingers and watches the identified tooth while the patient goes through the same movements. Fremitus is graded as:

I   movement felt but not visible

II   just visibly perceptible movement

III distinct visible movement.

The operator should record the tooth (teeth) involved, the grade of fremitus and whether fremitus occurs in intercuspal position, excursive movements or both. This whole screening process takes only a few seconds, but the presence of grade II or III fremitus is a strong indicator for the need for a detailed occlusal examination.

Special examinations

What radiographs?

Over the years, the criteria for minimum necessary radiographs has changed and evolved from a period of rigid dogma, where each discipline had its own required radiographs, through a period where sadly what was paid for by third parties became the norm. Now, hopefully, we have reached a more patient-focused era, when the findings of an initial clinical examination, combined with the full consideration of the chief complaint and history, establish what radiographs are the minimum necessary to provide the supplementary information needed to reach a full diagnosis and develop treatment plan options.

It should go without saying that it is not good practice to prescribe a standard series of radiographs for a new patient prior to carrying out a proper clinical examination. Not only does it fail to customise the radiographs taken to the individual patient's needs, but it also gives the impression of a conveyor belt approach to the more discerning new patient. This is certainly not a desirable impression to give, even before the patient meets the dentist.

What do we need to see? A fundamental question, which is not always asked when radiographs are taken, is what do we need to see? Among the essential pieces of information that can only be seen on radiograph are:

- the depth of penetration of clinically detectable areas of enamel decalcification
- where clinical caries is evident, its proximity to the pulp
- bone topography where significant periodontal probing depth is present
- the root length and apices of all teeth that may potentially act as abutments for fixed or removable prostheses
- the status of any edentulous area where tooth replacement is being considered: it is essential to be aware of the presence of any retained roots, unerupted teeth and (if implants are being considered as an option) the height of bone above major anatomic structures
- the proximity of large existing restorations to the pulp and, where there is a suggestion of a previous pulp exposure, the state of the apex of the tooth
- the apices of all teeth with previous root canal fillings
- the root length, bone support and status of periodontal ligament space on all teeth displaying increased mobilities and/or fremitus.

It should be noted that all of these indications are contingent on findings from the initial clinical examination, and again this emphasises the need for a clinical examination preceding the decision on necessary radiographs. The patient's history may well reveal that recent films have been taken elsewhere. At the very least, the dentist should call to clarify the types of view taken and these should be requested if pertinent to present needs. Only where urgent relief of pain is required, should an additional radiograph be taken when a recent view already exists. It may well be necessary to have the patient sign a release before the previous radiographs can be forwarded.

The sequence of the examination visit should allow for initial history taking and clinical examination, followed by the taking of the necessary films (delegated to an auxiliary where training and legislation permits), and development of tentative treatment options that will be refined after the radiographs have been processed. When an auxiliary is able to take the radiographs, it gives the dentist valuable 'thinking' time to

assimilate the initial findings and prepare for the second phase of the examination. While this will obviously not be necessary in more straightforward cases, it can be invaluable when the patient presents with more complex problems.

A case for vertical bitewings The bitewing radiograph has long been the workhorse of general dental practice, where the primary focus has traditionally been on detection and treatment of caries. Because it has been recommended as the primary screening radiograph in caries detection, and again because of the compartmentalisation of teaching, the overall diagnostic value of bitewings in detecting other pathology is often overlooked. Figure 2.19 shows not only interproximal contacts but also significant horizontal bone loss distal to 1-7, 2-7 likely related to wisdom tooth extraction. There is, however, a limit to the extent of bone visible on the standard horizontal bitewing, and for this reason the clinician should consider use of vertical bitewings as a standard screening tool in primary care.

Several studies show that, in a complete posterior dentition, it is necessary to take four bitewings rather than two to identify all interproximal caries. Single films will miss between 20 and 30% of lesions detected with bilateral double films, as a result of overlap and incomplete field of view. A series of four vertical bitewings will show considerably more of the bone support of the teeth while still providing all necessary information on interproximal and occlusal caries.

Panoramic radiographs Since their introduction, over 30 years ago, panoramic radiographs have gone through several periods of being more or less in favour. Their greatest value is likely in the partially edentulous patient where various options in tooth replacement are being considered. A traditional full mouth series of periapical radiographs often does not fully expose the edentulous areas or the position of several major structures such as inferior dental canals and maxillary sinuses. With improvements in panoramic technology and as endosseous implants have become a realistic treatment option in the general practice setting, the panoramic view has re-emerged as an invaluable screening radiograph in more complex cases.

Where multiple problems, including edentulous areas, are present, the panoramic radiograph is often the most versatile screening X-ray, providing full mouth information with limited radiation exposure in

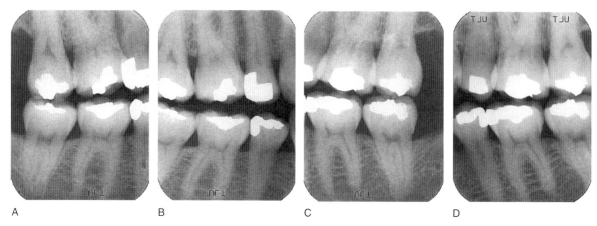

A   B   C   D

Figure 2.19 A set of vertical bitewing radiographs. These enable checking for interproximal caries and also have the ability to identify subgingival calculus and significant horizontal and vertical bone loss. There is a limit to the extent of bone visible on the standard horizontal bitewing.

a relatively short time frame. While it may take over 20 minutes to take, process and mount a full series of paralleling periapical films, a panoramic film, often supplying more information, can generally be taken and returned to chairside within 5 minutes, with less total radiation to the patient.

Digital radiography

The advent of practical digital radiography has been a significant step forward in efficient assembly of diagnostic data. It is now feasible, with less radiation than an equivalent conventional radiograph, to view the image in real time on a chairside computer screen, and this can then be printed as required. At present, there are some limitations to this technique: the quality of the image is generally of a somewhat lesser quality than a conventional radiograph; there is some difficulty with most of the present available systems in taking truly parallel long-cone films; and with most systems there is an enlargement factor that makes measuring for endodontics and implant planning difficult if not impossible.

At present, it would appear that digital radiography is most appropriate where an approximation of information is required quickly. Consequently, situations such as working length determination and other inter-mediate films in endodontics and rapid assessment of dental emergencies would seem to be the most useful applications of this exciting advance.

Study models: Diagnostic casts

There are limits to the information that can be gathered from a clinical and radiographic examination. Access limits visual assessment of tooth-to-tooth contact to only the buccal perspective, while radiographs are essentially two-dimensional representations of a three-dimensional situation, with all the limitations that this presents.

Study models, either hand held or mounted on some form of articulator, go some way to reduce these limitations and are indicated as follows:

- unmounted study casts (Fig. 2.20)
  — to assess static interarch relationships
  — to assess single arch problems such as pontic spaces
  — simple orthodontic assessment of intact dentitions
  — to record recession, wear facets, abrasion, etc.

- mounted casts on a hinge articulator (Fig. 2.21)
  — to assess static interarch relations where insufficient teeth are present to allow predictable hand-held interarch articulation
  — when a few teeth are to be replaced by a bridge or implant within an acceptable occlusal scheme
  — when a static diagnostic wax up is required

- mounted study casts on a semi-adjustable articulator (Fig. 2.22)

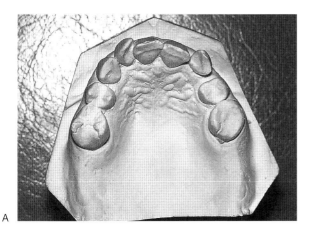

A

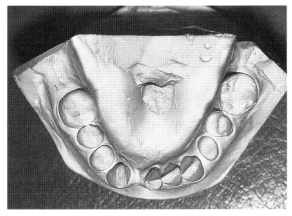

B

Figure 2.20 Unmounted upper (A) and lower (B) study casts are often sufficient to assess static interarch relationships, single arch problems such as pontic spaces, simple orthodontic assessment and to record recession or wear facets abrasion.

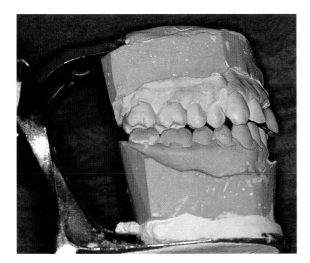

Figure 2.21 Study models mounted on a hinge articulator can be used to assess the situation in patients with relative simple problems.

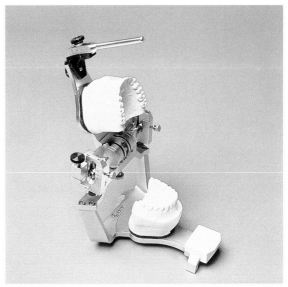

Figure 2.22 By use of a semiadjustable articulator with models mounted using a facebow and lateral check bites, the dentist can reproduce jaw movements and assess the effects of alterations to the occlusal vertical dimension (see Fig. 2.25). It is also possible to carry out trial occlusal adjustments on the models.

— where any major restorative dentistry is a likely treatment option
— where a change in vertical dimension is likely to be necessary
— where a significant discrepancy in intercuspal position (ICP) or retruded contact position (RCP) has been identified in association with some occlusal pathology.

There is in some circles a form of elitism based on always mounting casts on a semi-adjustable articulator. While this is often appropriate in more complex cases, it is certainly overkill where relatively simple restorative treatment at the presenting vertical dimension is planned. 'Always' and 'never' are seldom appropriate adverbs to qualify any dental procedure.

A diagnostic wax-up is an invaluable aid in planning both bridgework and implant-based restorations. It also allows the dentist to convey to the patient what is and is not feasible in the management of their problems. Patient C was unhappy with anterior aesthetics and had significant attrition and repeated fracture of an anterior bridge (Fig. 2.23). The first step was to confirm that she could tolerate an increased vertical dimension by the use (for 12 hours a day over several weeks) of an

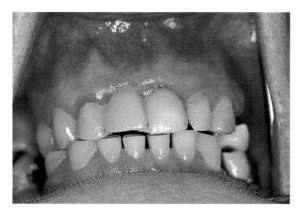

Figure 2.23 Patient C: the use of a diagnostic wax-up. This patient is unhappy with anterior aesthetics and had significant attrition and repeated fracture of an anterior bridge.

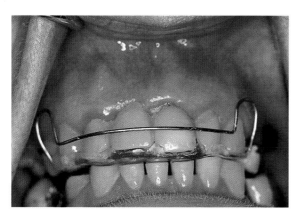

Figure 2.24 Initial assessment that Patient C could tolerate an increased vertical dimension, through wearing an anterior bite plane at an increased vertical dimension for several weeks.

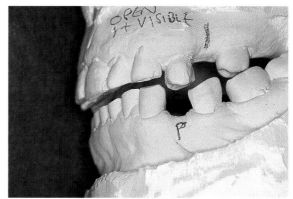

A

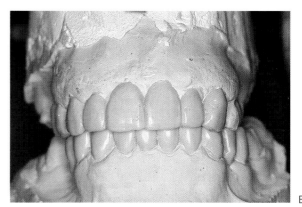

B

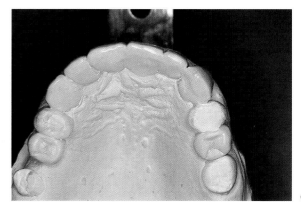

C

Figure 2.25 Study casts for Patient C based on the new vertical dimension.

anterior bite plane (Fig. 2.24). A diagnostic wax-up was then developed on a semi-adjustable articulator at the vertical established by the appliance (Fig. 2.25). The study casts were opened to the tested occlusal vertical dimension on a semi-adjustable articulator, and a diagnostic wax-up was carried out to allow the operator to assess occlusal relations at the new vertical and to allow the patient to see and approve a preview of the final treatment outcome. With the patient's approval the dentist could then proceed to a composite and non-precious alloy provisional restoration (Fig. 2.26).

Where appropriate a potential restoration can be placed on a stabilised denture try in base to allow the patient to preview the effect of tooth replacement in their own mouth. Patient D was unsure whether to replace two or three missing upper posterior teeth with an implant-supported restoration. By previewing the possible result with a simple denture wax-up (Fig. 2.27) she decided on three teeth. This was then taken to completion using the wax-up tooth position as a guide to implant placement (Fig. 2.28). The final result is close to the preview wax-up (Fig. 2.29). More importantly, this is a tangible form of informed consent.

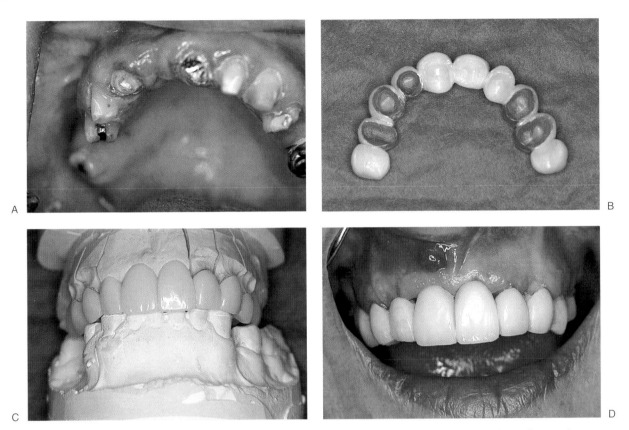

Figure 2.26 Once Patient C had approved the restoration, the teeth were prepared (A) and a non-precious alloy and composite provisional bridge made (B) copying the approved diagnostic wax-up (C). Teeth 1-2 and 2-1 were replaced by immediate implants.

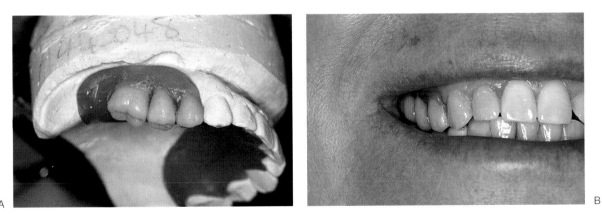

Figure 2.27 Patient D: the use of a simple denture wax-up to allow the patient to chose between two and three teeth in a restoration. Provided this can be reproduced in the final restoration, and the procedures and risks are explained in detail, the dentist has obtained informed consent.

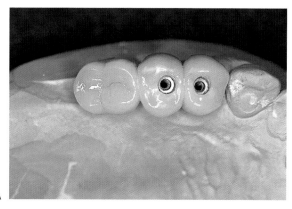
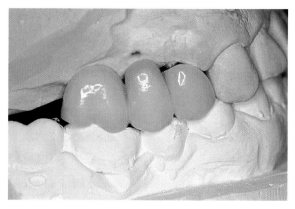

A   B

Figure 2.28 An implant-supported cantilever bridge is fabricated corresponding to the tooth position approved by Patient D on the wax-up.

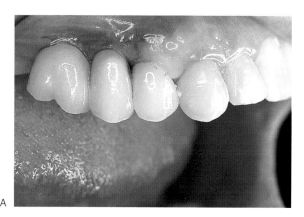
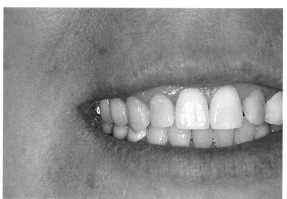

A   B

Figure 2.29 The definitive restoration is inserted and meets Patient D's expectations.

By careful removal and repositioning of individual teeth, it can also be possible to preview the effects of minor orthodontic tooth movement. The use of study casts is discussed in more detail in the section on occlusal objectives in Chapter 4.

Assessment of oral habits

In order to appreciate fully the factors contributing to dental problems, it is important to identify any repetitive habits that influence the dentition. Abrams classifies habits into:

- tooth to tooth habits: clenching, grinding, doodling, etc.

- tooth to oral musculature habits: cheek biting, tongue thrust, lip biting, etc.

- tooth to foreign object habits: thumb sucking, nail biting, pipe or pen biting, etc.

Tooth to tooth habits

Bruxing forces can be up to 20 times greater than normal chewing forces. While clenching may be directed along the long axis of teeth and only serve to transfer forces to temporomandibular joints and/or muscles, grinding forces are likely to damage the teeth or periodontium. Figure 2.30 shows a patient with a combined severe grinding habit with loss of posterior

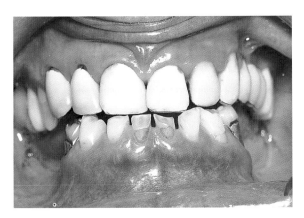

Figure 2.30 A severe grinding habit combined with loss of posterior teeth and opposing porcelain restorations has resulted in severe attrition of lower anterior teeth and loss of occlusal vertical dimension.

teeth and opposing porcelain restorations. The result is severe attrition of lower anterior teeth, as well as loss of occlusal vertical dimension.

Tooth to oral musculature habits

The repetitive nature of tooth to oral musculature habits can significantly influence tooth position. They are also often seen as secondary developments of other habits and unfavourable treatment outcomes. The patient in Figure 2.31 has an anterior open bite resulting from a long-standing thumb-sucking habit. In order to achieve a seal during swallowing, she has now developed an anterior tongue thrust. It is likely that, even if the thumb sucking ceases, the tongue thrust will prevent the open bite from correcting without active orthodontic treatment. The patient in Figure 2.32 has worn a mandibular orthopedic repositioning appliance (MORA) for several months. This has resulted not only in a posterior open bite but also a lateral tongue thrust, which is now preventing compensatory posterior eruption to re-establish posterior contact. It has been the author's experience that these appliances often cause such problems.

Tooth to foreign object habits

In addition to thumb sucking (see Fig. 2.31), patients can also alter occlusal relations with various other habits. The patient shown in Figure 2.33 has an acquired anterior open bite and a widening diastema between teeth 3-3 and 3-2. This has been caused by an almost incessant fingernail-biting habit, where the

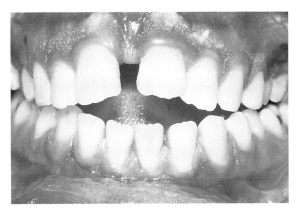

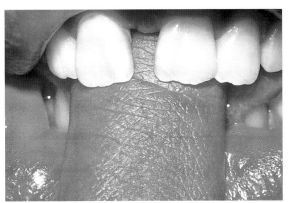

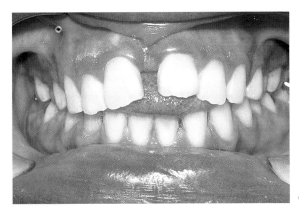

Figure 2.31 Tooth to oral musculature habit secondary to a tooth to foreign object habit. (A) This 20-year-old patient has an anterior open bite. Mamilons are still present on all incisors. (B) The patient still has a thumb-sucking habit, present since infancy, which has prevented full eruption of the incisors. (C) In order to create an anterior seal during swallowing an anterior tongue thrust is present.

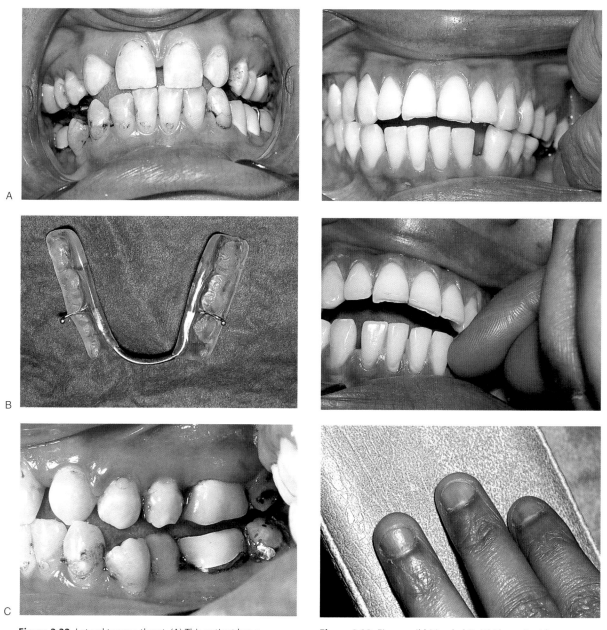

A

B

C

A

B

C

Figure 2.32 Lateral tongue thrust. (A) This patient has a bilateral posterior open bite. Only anterior teeth contact in 'intercuspal position'. (B) The mandibular orthopaedic repositioning appliance that led to the development of the tongue thrust habit. (C) Because of the bilateral posterior open bite, the patient has acquired a bilateral tongue thrust during swallowing. This will prevent posterior eruption and re-establishment of a stable posterior occlusion unless it can be controlled.

Figure 2.33 Fingernail-biting habit. (A) The patient has an anterior open bite and a widening diastema between teeth 3-3 and 3-2. (B) She admits to a fingernail-biting habit of long standing, placing each finger in turn adjacent to the lower diastema. (C) Examination of her fingernails reveals them to be severely bitten down. Note the dry wrinkled nature of the fingers resulting from constant exposure to saliva.

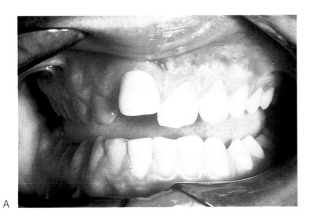

A

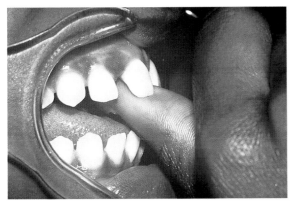

B

Figure 2.34 Finger-sucking habit. (A) This 19-year-old patient presented with the upper left central incisor severely proclined and with a grade 2 mobility. (B) The finger-sucking habit, which has caused the labial movement of the incisor.

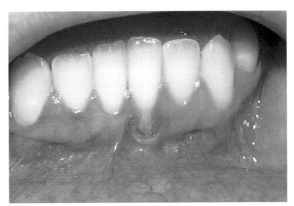

Figure 2.35 Repeated root scratching causing a localised area of recession.

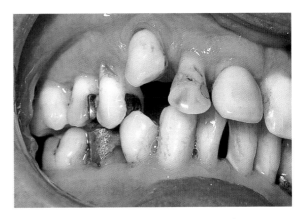

Figure 2.36 A pipe-holding habit has led to buccal movement of the upper right canine.

fingers are placed in turn into the space between 3-2 and 3-3. The patient has also developed an anterior disc displacement and myofascial pain.

The patient in Figure 2.34 has caused localised labial movement of the left central incisor by a **finger-sucking** habit focused on this one tooth. Repeated **root scratching** of an area of sensitivity by the patient in Figure 2.35 has resulted in considerable recession and worsening sensitivity. This patient was referred for a gingival graft to correct a localised area of recession on a lower incisor. During the consultation, it was noted that she had a habit of scratching the sensitive area of the root. Although she was initially unaware of this habit, she soon acknowledged it and it took over a year before the patient and author were confident the habit had been controlled. The grafting procedure had to be postponed until the habit was definitely controlled. Figure 2.36 shows the result of a

pipe-holding habit in a 55-year-old university professor who had smoked a pipe for over 30 years, habitually holding it in the right canine area. This has resulted in the labial movement of the upper canine. Based on the patient's history, the tooth had been in this position for many years, and clinically the tooth was solid and periodontally healthy. It had reached a position of equilibrium between pipe, lip and tongue and had little mobility.

WHEN SHOULD A DENTIST COMMUNICATE WITH THE PHYSICIAN?

As the combination of more effective dentistry and medicine produces an ageing dentate population, dentists will increasingly find themselves treating older patients with complex medical histories and who are often taking several medications. The rapid increase in the number of different prescription drugs in use makes it more likely that patients will present using medicines with which the dentist is not familiar. Several other aspects of the patient's history, and particularly when the history is unclear, may prompt the dentist to communicate with the general medical practitioner. Among these are when:

- the patient is unable to complete the medical history
- the patient cannot provide the name of a prescription drug they are taking
- the dentist identifies something that needs medical attention
- the patient presents with a medical situation that may need special treatment considerations
- it is unclear if the patient is fit for elective surgical procedures.

Although many physicians will provide necessary information in response to a telephone enquiry, this may well infringe on patient confidentiality, and it is generally best to have the patient sign a simple release form (see the Appendix) and to write formally to the physician outlining the reason for your enquiry (see the Appendix). This also has the benefit of documenting your request and the written response within the patient records.

When a patient presents with pain and immediate treatment is indicated, a telephone contact is most practical and, where the physician is hesitant to break confidentiality, the patient may be put on the line to give oral consent. All verbal communications should be written up in the patient's records.

3

The problem list: making sense of data

It is of the highest importance in the art of detection to recognize out of a number of facts, which are incidental and which are vital.

Sherlock Holmes: Sir Arthur Conan Doyle (1859–1930)

If the dentist can generally take a good history and assemble adequate diagnostic data, how can this be developed into an effective treatment plan? Most dental school records assemble diagnostic data in an almost random order, in various parts of the patient's chart. The student is then expected to develop a rational treatment plan from this convoluted data set. Even when data are assembled in a reasonably ordered, rational manner, it is not uncommon at the end of this process to be instructed to 'now assemble the treatment plan', with little if any guidance as to how this is achieved.

This is the worst of all possible worlds, since it guides the students through the largely mechanical process of recording relatively objective data but abandons them in the much more complex process of making sufficient sense of the data to develop treatment options. More damagingly, it gives the subliminal message that 'the data are the treatment plan', and can produce a plan that is no more than a list of fillings, treated in isolation rather than in the overall context of the patient's problems and desires.

On graduation, dentists generally associate with an experienced practitioner and use the record charts that are already in use in the practice. Practice forms are usually much shorter and simpler than those used in dental school, but this is often taken to a simplistic level, with little space for anything beyond a basic caries and periodontal charting. In many cases, these forms are developed by health service or insurance company bureaucrats, more for their administrative convenience than for the clinician's effective use. The classical format for history taking outlined in Chapter 2 is seldom accommodated in these forms developed by third parties.

While these records are generally adequate for the younger patient with an intact dentition, they are seldom sufficient to record the pertinent information for a patient with more complex problems. It is, therefore, often particularly difficult to review the pertinent findings in an organised way and in conjunction with radiographs and study casts.

DEVELOPING A PROBLEM LIST

The problem-oriented record was first developed for use in medicine in the early 1970s and was adapted for dentistry within a few years. This approach has been so successful, both as a teaching tool and as an effective way of delivering care, that over half the world's medical schools now used a problem-based curriculum, with a problem-oriented record at the heart of its clinical component.

Fundamental to the problem-oriented record is the use of a problem list. This has proven beneficial in simple treatment plans and is invaluable in complex treatment planning. To consider this properly, it is essential to define the terms involved.

*A **problem** is a finding (sign or symptom) that requires a separate course of action.*

Hence a problem can be very site specific, such as isolated caries on the buccal and occlusal of tooth 1-6, which may require two separate fillings, or it can be much more general, such as chronic gingivitis involving all teeth, requiring scaling, polishing and oral hygiene instruction.

In Figure 3.1, the three carious lesions on the buccal of teeth 4-3, 4-4 and 4-5 require three separate fillings and so are three separate problems. The gingivitis in Figure 3.2 is generalised to almost all teeth, and so one course of action, scaling, polishing and oral hygiene instruction, is required for the whole mouth. If, as in this case, mouthbreathing is identified as contributing to the anterior part of the gingivitis, it should be listed as another separate problem.

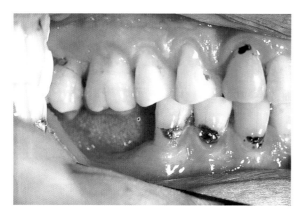

Figure 3.1 The caries on the buccal of teeth 4-3, 3-4 and 4-5 should be listed as three separate problems since they will need three separate actions (fillings) to address them. The missing molars are also a problem, which may or may not be addressed in the present course of treatment.

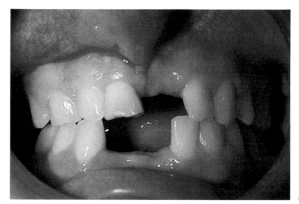

A

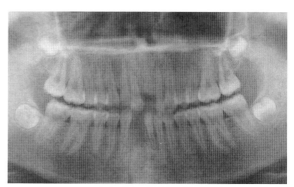

B

Figure 3.3 A 16-year-old patient (T.D.) after a major car accident. (A) Tooth 2-1 has been fractured beyond repair; tooth 1-1 has been reimplanted, and several other upper teeth are displaced and non-vital. Two lower incisors 4-1 and 4-2 have been lost and tooth 3-1 was avulsed, reimplanted but later lost. (B) An orthopantomogram taken at the time of the accident showed severely fractured 2-1, missing 4-1 and 4-2 as well as displaced and fractured 1-1 and 3-1. Note also developing wisdom teeth.

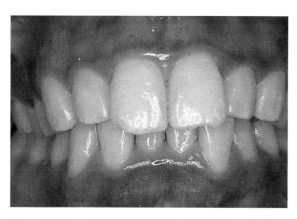

Figure 3.2 Generalised gingivitis is identified in this patient's mouth. Although this involves virtually all teeth, it is only *one* problem, since one course of action will address the problem for all teeth.

A problem may relate to the patient's medical history, for example a history of rheumatic fever is a problem, and antibiotic prophylaxis is the action required to address this. A problem may be based on time restraints of a job or access difficulty because the patient lives in a remote location. Equally, a problem may also relate to the patient's desires and expectations or even their ease of access to treatment.

An example of a problem list

These principles are applied to a case of medium complexity in the following section.

The 16-year-old patient (T.D.) in Figure 3.3 was involved in a major car accident. Aside from other injuries, tooth 2.1 was fractured beyond repair; tooth 1-1 had been reimplanted, and several other upper teeth were displaced and non-vital. Two lower incisors 4-1 and 4-2 were lost and tooth 3-1 was displaced and partly repositioned. Initial X-ray film showed the extent of the damage (Fig. 3.3B). Subsequently root canal treatment and orthodontic realignment were completed (Fig. 3.4A,B). Tooth 1-1 had a short root, possible root resorption and had been reimplanted; its long-term prognosis was not good and it should certainly not be a terminal bridge abutment. Tooth 3-1 exhibited root resorption, had become non-vital and had an apical area. Since adjacent teeth had no damage, a bridge, is contraindicated. Tooth 3-1 had a

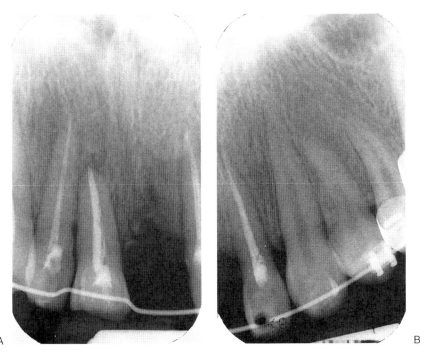

A   B

Figure 3.4 Root canal treatment and orthodontic repositioning. (A) Teeth 1-2 and 1-1: note the short root and possible early root resorption on tooth 1-1. (B) Tooth 2-2: because a root-treated lateral is not an ideal terminal abutment for an extensive bridge, especially if tooth 1-1 is eventually lost, extension of a future bridge to the canine should be considered.

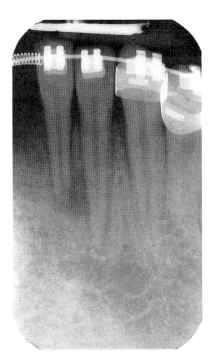

Figure 3.5 Tooth 3-1 showing apical resorption and mobility.

poor prognosis and complicated possible implant treatment, and so it was decided to extract this tooth.

At the time of treatment planning, orthodontics had been completed, and the patient's chief complaint was the compromised appearance and her fear of complex treatment. The patient at this point was almost 18 years of age and appeared fully grown; consequently, implant replacement was feasible and a final restorative plan could be made. Various other clinical findings were present and may also require attention (Fig. 3.6). As the situation becomes more complex, a list of problems is developed (Table 3.1). At this stage, the order in which problems are listed does not matter.

> A **problem list** *is a numbered list of identified problems, with each problem listed on a separate line, and with a column to the right allowing classification into 'active' and 'inactive' problems (Table 3.1).*

Each problem is expressed at the clinician's level of knowledge. This makes the use of a problem list as applicable to a first year dental student as to an experienced clinician. By opening-up communications

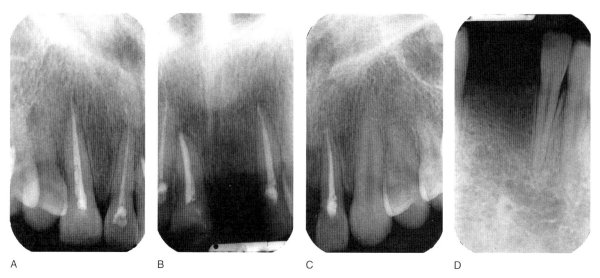

A   B   C   D

Figure 3.6 The radiographs before a final restorative treatment for Patient T.D. Orthodontics has been completed, satisfactory endodontics was present on all non-vital teeth and the extraction site of 3-1 had healed.

Table 3.1 Problem list for Patient T.D.

Problem	Status (active/inactive)
1. Missing tooth 2-1	
2. Reimplanted tooth 1-1 with root resorption and/or short root	
3. Fractured tooth 1-1	
4. Fractured tooth 1-2	
5. Fractured tooth 2-2	
6. Missing teeth 3-1, 4-1, 4-2	
7. Loss of buccal plate in area of 2-1	
8. Unhappy with aesthetics	
9. Desire to avoid removable dentures	
10. Fearful of dental treatment	
11. Bilateral temporo-mandibular joint click	
12. Localised gingivitis	
13. Unerupted wisdom teeth	
14. Patient lives 250 miles from practice	

between neophyte clinician, expert and the patient, the problem list becomes a very robust teaching, communication and planning tool. The cervical brown lesion on the tooth in Figure 3.7 might be expressed as 'a brown mark' by the patient, 'recession above the crown' by the student and as 'exposed non-vital root due to recession' by the expert. It becomes clear that all parties are talking about the same thing, and hence communications between those with different skill levels is facilitated. The lower incisors in Figure 3.8 might be described as 'too short' by the patient, as 'worn down' by the student and as 'advanced attrition' by the expert. All would be acceptable on the initial problem list.

SEPARATING ACTIVE AND INACTIVE PROBLEMS

Having listed the problems, in any order, the dentist must now differentiate *active* problems and *inactive* problems:

- *an **active** problem is one that will be addressed within the present treatment plan*
- *an **inactive** problem is a variance from the norm, which is to be monitored but does not need active treatment within the present treatment plan.*

It is, therefore, possible for the same situation to be an active problem in one patient while being inactive in another. A midline diastema may be the patient's chief complaint and obviously an active problem (Fig. 3-9), or it may be something that the patient is happy to accept, and hence an inactive problem (Fig. 3-10). The 22-year-old patient shown in Figure 3.9 presented with a chief complaint of 'I hate my teeth, I never smile'. When questioned, she identified

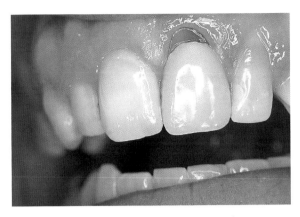

Figure 3.7 This patient presented with recession above a crown on a non-vital tooth.

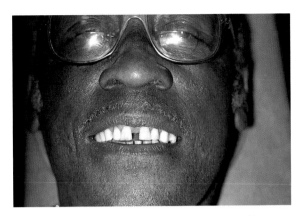

Figure 3.10 A midline diastema that is an inactive problem.

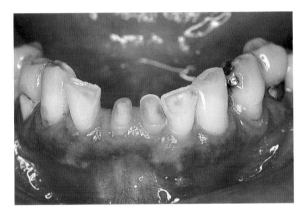

Figure 3.8 Worn lower incisors.

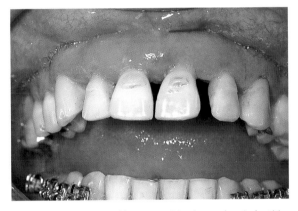

Figure 3.11 A 38-year-old woman with advanced periodontitis and flaring of her upper anterior teeth. She stated that the teeth used to be together with no spacing and this must be considered to be an active problem because the situation is unstable.

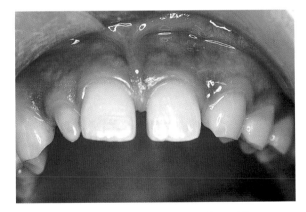

Figure 3.9 A midline diastema that is an active problem.

the midline diastema to be one of the aspects of her anterior teeth that she did not like. Although all anterior teeth are free of caries and periodontal problems, this clearly must be considered to be an active problem. By comparison the 55-year-old man shown in Figure 3.10 stated that his midline diastema had been the same for as long as he can remember. He felt that the space was 'part of me' and had no desire to change it. The teeth are free of caries and periodontal disease and so this diastema should be listed as an inactive problem. If, however, the diastema was increasing because of progressive periodontal bone loss and lack of a stable posterior occlusion, then it will be an active problem, even if the patient is unaware of it and is unconcerned about its appearance (Fig. 3.11). In this last situation, the periodontal disease and the lack of posterior occlusion are also likely to be active problems. In other words, the diastema is unlikely to be treated effectively unless all three active problems are addressed.

Table 3.2 Problem list for Patient T.D.

Problem	Status (A, active; I, inactive)
1. Missing tooth 2-1	A
2. Reimplanted tooth 1-1 with root resorption and/or short root	A
3. Fractured tooth 1-1	A
4. Fractured tooth 1-2	A
5. Fractured tooth 2-2	A
6. Missing teeth 3-1, 4-1, 4-2	A
7. Loss of buccal plate and soft tissue in area of 2-1	A
8. Unhappy with aesthetics	A
9. Desire to avoid removable dentures	A
10. Fearful of dental treatment	A
11. Bilateral temporomandibular joint click	I[a]
12. Localised gingivitis	A
13. Unerupted wisdom teeth	I[b]
14. Patient lives 250 miles from practice	A

[a]Since the clicks are reducing in frequency and severity it is decided to monitor both the joint noises clinically and the condyles radiographically.
[b]Wisdom teeth are in favourable position and it is decided to monitor their eruption.

An example of active and inactive problems

Returning to the patient T.D. (Figs 3.3–3.6), the problem list (Table 3.1) can be divided into active and inactive problems (Table 3.2). Temporomandibular joint (TMJ) radiographs (Fig. 3.12) showed possible bone changes in the left condyle. As there was no pain on palpation and clicks were becoming less frequent, it was decided to monitor this situation.

THE PROBLEM–BASED TREATMENT PLAN FOR ACTIVE PROBLEMS

A problem-based treatment plan is a logical sequence of therapy that *addresses all the active problems* and that plans for future *monitoring of presently inactive problems.*

By using a cross-reference to the original problem list, the clinician can confirm that none of the active problems has been forgotten. This is generally done by listing the number of the problem addressed to the right of each item of treatment. Table 3.3 shows this approach applied to Patient T.D.

The use of intravenous sedation both allows management of the patient's anxiety and addresses the distance factor by allowing more to be achieved on each appointment. The treatment plan as outlined can then be carried to completion as planned (Figure 3.13). The earlier treatment after the accident involved root canal treatment and a reimplanted tooth (1-1). Consequently, the final bridge is cemented with a temporary cement so that, if tooth 1-1 is lost through resorption or any of the root canal-treated teeth develop a root fracture, the bridge can be easily converted and reused after extraction. While this is sensible forward planning in every case, it becomes especially important when, in an accident case with treatment paid for by a third party, future retreatment because of such a complication may be financially difficult or impossible for the patient.

Once a draft treatment plan has been developed, the dentist should refer to the problem list and confirm that all active problems have been addressed and that monitoring for inactive problems is planned. Chapter

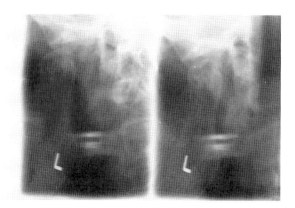

Figure 3.12 Temporomandibular radiographs of Patient T.D. indicating possible bone changes in the left condyle.

Table 3.3 Treatment plan for Patient T.D.

Treatment	Problem(s) addressed
1. Scale and polish	12
2. Oral hygiene instruction; especially flossing	12
3. Reassess oral hygiene and periodontal status	12
4. Intravenous conscious sedation for long appointments	10, 14
5. Temporary bridge from teeth 1-3 to 2-3	1, 2, 3, 4, 5, 8, 9
6. Connective tissue graft to augment 2-1 area	7
7. Place two mandibular titanium implants	6
8. Temporary lower partial denture	8
9. Cast metal posts and cores for teeth 1-3, 1-2, 1-, 2-2	3, 4 ,5
10. Expose implants and place healing abutments	6
11. Relieve and soft reline lower partial denture	8
12. Fabricate upper 6-unit bridge	1, 2, 3, 4, 5, 8, 9
13. Fabricate lower 3-unit implant bridge	6, 9
14. Annual implant/restorative/TMJ/wisdom tooth recall	All
15. Routine care with local general dentist	11, 12, 13, 14

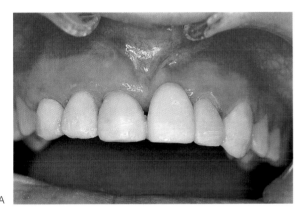
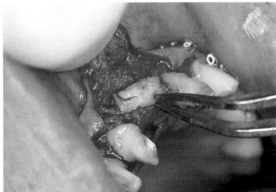
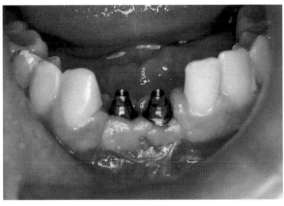
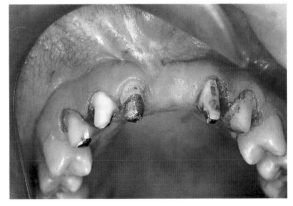

A   B   C   D

Figure 3.13 Final treatment for Patient T.D. (A) A 6-unit temporary bridge is in place. The pontic (tooth 2-1) was significantly longer cervically due to the loss of buccal place and soft tissue in the accident. After discussion with patient and parents it was decided to augment the area in order to establish symmetry (see Ch. 10). (B) A connective tissue graft was placed to augment the edentulous ridge. While this was ideal for tooth-supported bridgework, bone augmentation would be necessary if an implant was to be placed. (C) Two titanium implants have been placed and have integrated successfully. Abutments are in place prior to impression taking. (D) Cast metal post and cores have been placed and final impressions are taken. Note the successfully augmented ridge. *Continued*

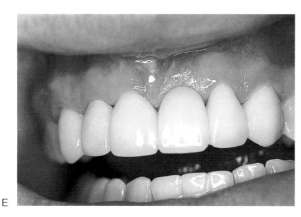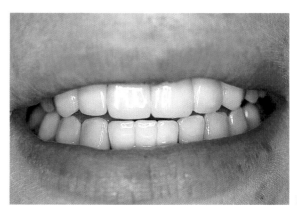

E   F

Figure 3.13, cont'd (E) A final porcelain bonded to gold alloy bridge is placed. (F) A final smile picture shows a satisfactory aesthetic result with a good long-term prognosis.

4 will address the logical development of a multi-disciplinary treatment plan, using the problem list as a facilitator.

SUMMARY

After assembling all pertinent data, following the approach outlined in Chapter 2, the clinician should:

1.   Develop a problem list

2.   Differentiate between *active* and *inactive* problems

3.   Develop a logical sequence of therapy that *addresses all the active problems* and which plans for future *monitoring of presently inactive problems*

4.   Review the problem list, to confirm that all active problems have been addressed in the treatment plan.

4 Developing treatment options: ideal and acceptable compromise plans

WHAT IS AN 'IDEAL' TREATMENT PLAN?

A course of action might be considered 'ideal' if it was best when all of the circumstances that prevail have been taken into consideration. To be more specific, a treatment plan would be considered ideal if it achieved the best possible long-term outcomes for the patient, while addressing all patient concerns and active problems, with the minimum necessary intervention.

The dentist should decide on what is the best treatment option to recommend, based on the current evidence base rather than on personal preferences or bias. What is the best available may differ from the best he can provide, and it may also differ from what is covered by third party payments. We have an obligation to offer referral where appropriate and to present patients with *all* reasonable options, not to prejudge what they are likely to be able to choose or can afford.

Overall circumstances may modify what is best, and the whole mouth must be considered rather than an individual tooth. Figure 4.1 shows a badly broken down tooth 2-4, with a non-vital pulp and significant undermining of the remaining tooth structure by

caries. In an intact arch, it might well be best to carry out a root canal treatment, followed by fabrication of a cast metal post and core and a porcelain or metal ceramic crown. Depending on the depth of caries, crown lengthening may also be required. If, however, the teeth on either side of tooth 2-4 are heavily filled, and would benefit from crowns in their own right, then possibly extraction and a 3-unit bridge would be best. It is also feasible that extraction and a partial denture could be the best option where a free end saddle is present on the other side of the arch. If sufficient bone was present, and the patient was fit for elective surgery, then implant-supported crowns may well be better than a denture in the latter situation. To treat the tooth in isolation, without considering these other aspects, is unlikely to result in optimum care. When a patient presents on an emergency basis with pain, insufficient time may be available to make a full assessment of the mouth and develop all treatment options. In these circumstances, a phased approach may be appropriate. This would involve first relieving the pain, preferably without taking an irreversible step such as extraction, then having the patient return for comprehensive examination and treatment planning. Provided pain is relieved effectively, this approach is likely to make a favourable impression on the patient, not only because of the effective relief of pain but also because of the more comprehensive approach taken to their overall dental care.

There are often situations when two or more very good options are available. In these circumstances, it is the dentist's obligation to present all of these options, outlining the 'pros' and 'cons' of each. Factors that must be discussed for each option include:

- likely longevity (this should be evidence-based)
- cost
- invasiveness/reversibility
- success rates (again, evidence-based)
- possible complications

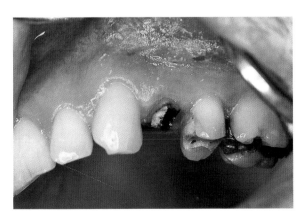

Figure 4.1 A badly broken down tooth 2-4, with a non-vital pulp and significant undermining of the remaining tooth structure by caries.

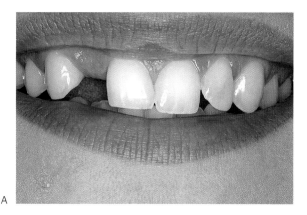

A

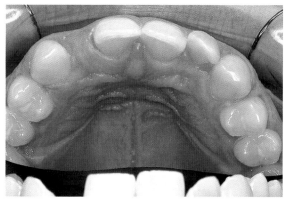

B

Figure 4.2 A single tooth space caused by loss of tooth 1-2.

- time involved, both total treatment time and number of visits
- influence on quality of life.

Let us consider the single incisor tooth space in Figure 4.2. Treatment options discussed may include:

- a single tooth implant
- a resin-retained bridge
- a 'conventional' 3-unit bridge
- a partial denture

These need to be considered in the light of the factors listed above. Although unlikely in this instance, the 'do nothing' option should always be discussed.

Provided the bone foundation is satisfactory, the **single tooth implant** has a high success rate (better than 95% in non-smokers); it has a higher initial cost than the other options and involves a longer treatment time with more visits, but it is likely to have the longest success rate. While it is invasive in terms of at least one surgical procedure, it is reversible to the

extent that the implant could be removed with minimal lasting damage and the adjacent teeth have not been touched. The most significant possible complication is implant failure, but surgical damage to adjacent teeth is also possible

A **resin-retained bridge** is likely to involve no surgery, has a good 3 to 5 year success rate but is less likely to last 10 years and is likely to be less costly than two of the other options. The most likely complication is debonding and this may, on occasion, lead to caries of an abutment tooth. It is a relatively non-invasive technique with limited removal of enamel and total treatment time is fairly short. While this approach may be considered a compromise in many patients, it may be the most appropriate in a young patient, used as a medium-term restoration until the patient has fully grown.

A 'conventional' **3-unit bridge** would also avoid surgery but does involve irreversible cutting down of abutment teeth, with a 20–25% risk of endodontic complications on one or other of these teeth. Other complications include caries, porcelain fracture and loss of retention with need for re-cementation. Various studies suggest a lifespan of 8 to 12 years, and initial costs are likely to be higher than either the partial denture or the resin-retained bridge.

A **partial denture** will be the least expensive option; it will generally be totally reversible, although rest seats and guide planes may be cut on adjacent teeth, and is likely to last at least 5 to 10 years. Possible complications include intolerance by the patient, alteration to phonetics and taste, soft tissue trauma leading to periodontal damage and the risk of caries if there is poor oral hygiene. Total treatment time will be short, with no need for local anaesthetic, but the compromised quality of life experienced by many denture wearers differentiates this from the other options.

If the dentist considers more than one of these options to be 'ideal' then the facts should be given to the patient, and they should make the final decision. More often the dentist considers one of these options to be 'ideal' and the others to be acceptable compromises.

Some apparently similar cases do not allow the same range of options. The patient shown in Figure 4.3 also has a single missing incisor (tooth 2-1). Because the edentulous space is 2 mm wider that the other central incisor, and there is a deep bite, the treatment options are more limited. A resin-retained bridge would have

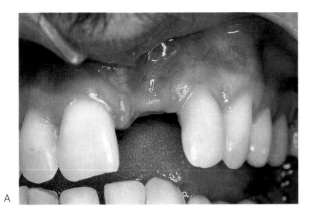

A

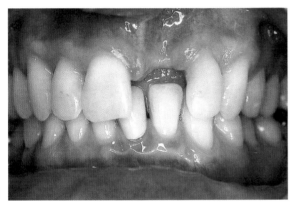

B

Figure 4.3 A single missing incisor (tooth 2-1) with more limited treatment options because the edentulous space is 2 mm wider that the other central incisor and there is a deep bite.

a limited prognosis and would involve a larger pontic or a significant diastema on one side; a conventional bridge would necessitate oversizing of at least the central incisors and a denture would risk fracture of the tooth from the base. 'Ideal' treatment is likely to be an implant-supported crown, with a conventional bridge, a partial denture and even a spring cantilever bridge as acceptable compromises.

WHAT COMPROMISES ARE ACCEPTABLE?

It is not always possible for the patient to proceed with the recommended ideal option. This is most often because of costs but can also on occasion be because of a time factor or because the patient has a bias against recommended treatment ('My friend had root canal treatment and still lost the tooth'). In most situations, there are reasonable alternatives to the recommended

ideal. These should be considered to be *acceptable compromises*.

For the patient shown in Figure 4.1, root canal treatment followed by a cast post core and crown may well be considered the ideal option. Acceptable compromises would include a preformed post and core system or a core build-up in amalgam or composite around a preformed post, or even dentine pins. It would also likely be acceptable to complete the root canal treatment and place a post or pin supported amalgam as the definitive restoration. It is, however, unrealistic to expect all of these compromises to fair as well or last as long as the ideal option. For this patient, the dentist could list the options as

- ideal: endodontics, cast post core and crown
- acceptable compromises
  — endodontics, preformed post core and crown
  — endodontics amalgam or composite build-up and crown
  — endodontics preformed post or pins and large amalgam filling.

It might also be considered acceptable to extract the tooth, leaving a space or replacing it with a conventional or resin-retained bridge or an implant-supported crown. It should be made very clear to the patient that a compromise option is just that: a compromise. When this is the patient's choice, the patient must be advised that they have to accept significantly more responsibility for this choice if and when deterioration occurs. However, when the patient agrees to the 'ideal' option, the dentist should be prepared to accept most of the responsibility for the outcome of this option.

If the dentist fails to offer all options, perhaps pre-judging the patient as 'not interested in' or 'not able to afford' ideal treatment, and proceeds to recommend only compromise choices, then the dentist must be prepared to accept full responsibility for whichever choice is made by the patient. There are no benefits and many potential problems when the patient is not given a full range of options.

When faced with complex problems and various treatment plan options, most patients will wonder, 'What will happen if I do nothing?' This is, however, not a question that is often asked. The dentist should try to preempt this question by including the 'do nothing' scenario in discussing treatment. Depending on the situation, this may involve likely tooth loss, overeruption, future pain and various other sequelae.

It is also likely to complicate or even negate some future treatment options, and this should be explained to the patient.

PROGNOSIS: HOW LONG WILL IT LAST?

It is obvious that different treatment approaches will not all have the same prognosis. Carrying forward the example above, it is likely that the ideal treatment option, well executed, is likely to last longer that the large amalgam filling. There is now a growing evidence base for the longevity of various restorative treatment procedures. It is not unreasonable for the patient to expect informed advice concerning the likely lifespan of each option from the practitioner recommending the various treatment choices.

Care must be taken to be sufficiently familiar with the relevant studies and to ensure that the method carried out by the dentist is consistent with that in the study. Most studies suggest a significantly higher long-term success with resin-retained bridges placed under rubber dam. If the dentist quotes these high success rates, he must be prepared to follow the same level of care throughout the procedure. Equally, the high long-term success rates in well-established implant systems cannot be extrapolated to new, less-proven systems. As well as following all specific stages in any recommended procedure, it is also important to allow sufficient time where this is integral to success. Most research on successful periodontal maintenance for patients with advanced periodontitis involves not only 3-monthly professional cleanings but also a full hour per visit for scaling, root planing and oral hygiene review. By advising 3-monthly maintenance but only allowing 20 or 30 minutes, the dentist should not represent this as ideal treatment for the periodontally involved patient.

Since the dentist is ultimately responsible for the treatment provided, it is important to become familiar with the research evidence (or lack of it) supporting any new technique or material recommended by a sales representative or laboratory. General practice is not the appropriate setting for uncontrolled, un-consented research on new unproven materials or techniques.

It is misleading for a patient when the dentist uses expressions such as 'permanent' crowns, bridges or even cements. Although unintentionally, this implies that the restorations will last indefinitely and has been shown in some legislations to imply a guarantee. It is wiser to use terms such as long-term, medium-term and short-term restorations.

WORKING WITH SPECIALISTS: WHEN TO REFER

The dentist has an ethical obligation to inform the patient of the best option and, where necessary, to offer the choice of referral to a specialist colleague who may be better able to provide more advanced care. General medical practitioners have little problem in referring their patients to specialist colleagues where indicated, and yet many general dentists appear to feel it their right, or perhaps duty, to provide all treatment to their patient. While this was often feasible 50 or more years ago, increased treatment options and patient expectations, combined with an increasing litigenous environment, make this a naive and simplistic approach for the twenty-first century. It is both the sign of a mature general dentist and, often, an effective practice builder to offer patients the best of care by working with specialists when this is indicated.

WORKING WITH A HYGIENIST: EFFECTIVE DELEGATION

Many aspects of general dental care involve carrying out relatively simple, repetitive and, on occasion, time-consuming procedures. As a practice becomes busy, the dentist often develops an interest in, and derives more enjoyment and financial reward from, more advanced procedures, and there is a temptation to rush or limit the time spent on these more basic aspects of care. Since many of these simple procedures are fundamental to good dental practice, the quality of care provided is likely to decline. This trend is, on occasion, accelerated by third parties assigning relatively lower fees for these simple procedures, forcing the dentist to accept a lower hourly return if the appropriate time is taken.

While legislation on the range of duties allocated to dental hygienists varies from country to country and between states and provinces in North America, most parts of the world recognise dental hygienists as a fundamental part of the dental team. It is in everyone's interest that available time is used efficiently and when a procedure can be effectively delegated to an auxiliary, while maintaining the standard of care, this should be done. It allows the dentist to devote more time to the more advanced procedures for which he or she alone is trained, while removing the pressures of providing all aspects of care. It allows hygienists to use the full range of their training and it provides the patient with optimum care at an economic fee.

It is likely that, in future, there will be a steady increase in delegation of a range of basic dental procedures, and while this will free up the dentist's time for more advanced procedures, it will also require practice management skills not extensively taught in dental schools. Among procedures already delegated in various parts of the world are:

- taking and developing intraoral and extraoral radiographs
- impressions for study models, model pouring and trimming
- administration of infiltration local anaesthesia
- scaling, polishing and root planing
- oral hygiene instruction
- fissure sealing
- placement of rubber dam
- placement of linings and plastic fillings
- changing of root canal medicament
- fabrication and placement of temporary restorations
- placement of fixed orthodontic appliances (brackets and archwires).

In most of these areas, controlled blind studies have shown that there is no significant difference in the quality of care provided comparing dentists with appropriately trained auxiliaries. General dentists who do not use auxiliaries should ask themselves if they provide all aspects of these duties to a high level of care and, if not, should consider effective delegation of such duties as local legislation allows. It is over 200 years since Adam Smith identified the economic benefits of division of labour; even by the conservative standards of dentistry, the wholehearted adoption of effective delegation can only be beneficial for all members of the dental team as well as for all other stakeholders in the practise of dentistry.

ELECTIVE ENDODONTICS: IF IT IS GOING TO DIE, KILL IT

By their very nature, many crowns and bridge abutments are placed on teeth that have had several large restorations in the past. It is fundamental to the assessment of any tooth planned for a crown or bridge abutment that the dentist is aware of the pulp status and apical situation of the tooth. Hence a periapical radiograph is mandatory. Not only will it allow assessment of the apex of the tooth but it will also provide information on the present and potential crown to root ratio, the depth of existing restorations and the size and position of the pulp. It also allows assessment of the adequacy of any existing root canal fillings. Electric and/or thermal pulp vitality testing is also strongly advised, particularly when any deep restoration is present.

There is good evidence that between 20 and 25% of teeth prepared for crowns will subsequently need root canal treatment. With this level of risk, it is necessary to inform the patient as part of the case presentation and treatment plan. There is also now considerable research showing that endodontics has its highest success rate when it is carried out *before* the development of a periapical radiolucency, and that endodontics re-treatment has a significantly lower success rate, even when carried out to high standards, than initial treatment. Hence there is a sound argument for early endodontics intervention in teeth that are at high risk of future periapical pathology. This does not mean that every tooth being crowned or used as a bridge abutment should have endodontics. It does, however, make it fundamental that the dentist should assess all such teeth on their individual merits, reach an evidence-based decision of the need for endodontics and communicate to patients the risks and benefits of elective endodontics.

The patient shown in Figure 4.4 was found to have an acute pulpitis, which had developed during crown preparation of a tooth. The chances of pulp recovery were remote. Since this tooth was an important abutment in a major reconstruction (see Figs 4.5–4.8, below), endodontics was carried out immediately, with conservative access preserving as much tooth structure as possible. If endodontics had been attempted after bridge cementation, the potential complications of attempting root canal treatment through the completed crown would include unnecessary destruction of tooth structure, loss of retention and a dissatisfied patient seeing a hole cut in a recently completed bridge. It is inevitable that more tooth structure would be destroyed finding the root canal and there would be a significant risk of later loss of retention. Elective endodontics was chosen and the bridge placed subsequently (Fig. 4.4C); to the author's knowledge it was functioning well at least 13 years later.

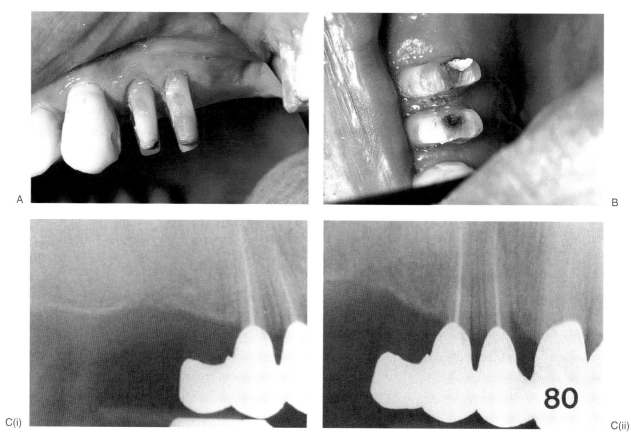

Figure 4.4 Acute pulpitis observed in a key abutment tooth during crown preparation (A,B). Elective endodontics is indicated. (C) Endodontics was completed and the bridge is in place.

BASIC OCCLUSAL OBJECTIVES: WHAT WORKS?

Chapter 2 discussed occlusal screening to determine when more detailed occlusal examination was necessary. When it has been decided that changes in the occlusion are necessary, then the dentist must have a clear picture in mind as to the therapeutic endpoint of treatment. Occlusion literature is complex, confusing and largely dogma based. Several different terms are often used to describe the same occlusal position, for example centric occlusion, intercuspal position, habitual occlusion and maximum intercuspation. There is, however, a general consensus within most occlusal philosophies as to what is considered a desirable endpoint of complex restorative care. This is often referred to as a **mutually protected occlusion** (Figs 4.5–4.7), which is so named because of its characteristics.

- The posterior teeth protect the anteriors when closing into maximum intercuspation by providing multiple simultaneous bilateral posterior contacts when the front teeth are just out of contact.

- The anterior teeth protect the posteriors during lateral and protrusive contacts by providing immediate disocclusion. This is achieved by a combination of incisal guidance discluding all posteriors in protrusion (Fig. 4.6), and canine guidance or group function (canine plus premolar buccal cusps) doing the same in lateral movements, allowing no contacts on the non-working side (Fig. 4.7).

- There is a coincidence of the intercuspal position with the retruded contact position.

While all of these features are not achievable in every complex treatment plan, it is the author's experience that the closer the clinician comes to

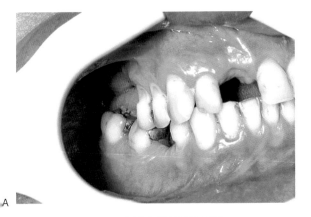

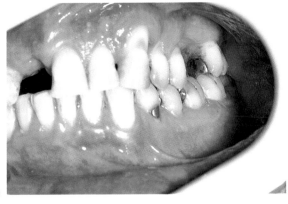

A

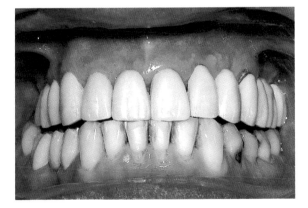

B

Figure 4.5 Patient D with a desire to eliminate a partial denture and with mutilated dentition, moderate to advanced periodontitis and recent tooth loss.

Figure 4.6 Incisal guidance immediately discludes all posterior teeth in protrusive movement.

achieving all of these objectives, the less one is likely to have future problems; conversely the more these principles are disregarded, the greater is the risk of future complications. The achievement of a mutually

protected occlusion is illustrated in Figures 4.5–4.8. Patient D was 50 years old and presented with a mutilated dentition, recent tooth loss caused by periodontal disease, moderate to advanced periodontitis with increased mobilities on the upper arch and a desire to eliminate his partial denture. Figures 4.6 and 4.7 show how the mutually protected occlusion was achieved and Figure 4.8 shows the final bridgework.

When part of the mutually protected occlusion is established by the use of a removable partial denture, the clinician must consider the nature of the occlusion at night when the partial is generally left out. This is the time when increased occlusal forces from clenching and grinding are most common, and, particularly in the presence of veneers or post crowns and when teeth are periodontally compromised, consideration should be given to some form of night protection. This may involve wearing the denture at night after appropriate oral hygiene has been carried out, but most commonly it is provided by fabrication of some form of **hard acrylic nightguard** or **splint** (Fig. 4.9). When anterior guidance cannot be developed during the day, as in some class 2 occlusions, an effort to establish it at night in a night splint will usually provide the necessary long-term protection for the teeth and restorations.

In a patient with no denture experience, where restoration of the posterior occlusion is dependent on successfully wearing a distal extension partial denture, it is wise to have the patient prove that they can cope with this before embarking on any high-risk anterior restorations. Both veneers and post crowns fall into this category. While these are generally predictable restorations in an intact dentition, they are much more prone to problems in the absence of a posterior occlusion. It is poor practice to provide these types of anterior restoration unless it is first established that the patient is able and willing to accept the restoration of a posterior occlusion, and provision has been made for some form of night time protection.

The shortened dental arch

Hand in hand with the attempt to develop a mutually protected occlusion, the general dentist should always ask how many teeth the patient actually needs. Although historically, the preservation or replacement of 28 teeth was considered desirable in every case, recent research has indicated that this is not always necessary and the concept of the shortened dental arch

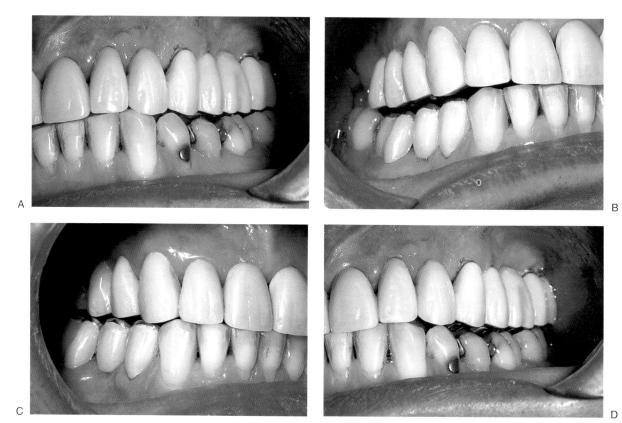

A

B

C

D

Figure 4.7 Canine guidance. Movement to the left side (A) discludes all teeth posterior to the canine as well as all teeth on the right (non-working) side (B). Similarly, movement to the right side (C) discludes all teeth posterior to the canine as well as all teeth on the left (non-working) side (D).

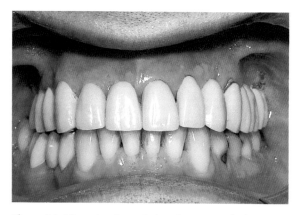

Figure 4.8 After extensive periodontal treatment, final bridgework for Patient D conforms to a mutually protected occlusion.

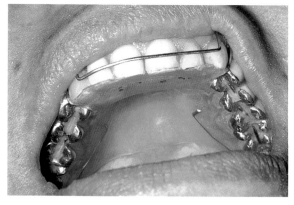

Figure 4.9 A hard acrylic nightguard.

initially proposed in the Netherlands has received wide acceptance. This generally requires:

- stable posterior contacts as far back as the first molar or second premolar provided there is a centric stop on the canines.
- a class 1 angle relationship
- all the above features of a mutually protected occlusion
- control of dental diseases on the remaining teeth.

It is considered more appropriate in older patients and where achievable may well negate the need for complex, expensive and often high-risk treatment on the more posterior teeth. Kayser (Kayser, 1981, 1994; Aukes et al., 1988) who has for many years been a leading advocate of this approach, cites the following criteria as being necessary for a shortened dental arch to be considered:

- progressive caries and periodontal disease confined mainly to the molars
- anterior and premolar teeth with favourable prognosis
- financial and other limitations to dental care.

He feels it is contraindicated in patients under 50 with:

- angle class III, severe angle class II or anterior open bite
- a marked reduction in alveolar bone support
- evidence of parafunction or abnormal wear for the patient's age
- pre-existing temporomandibular disorders.

The 57-year-old patient shown in Figure 4.10 was restored to a shortened dental arch after extensive periodontal treatment and the earlier loss of many

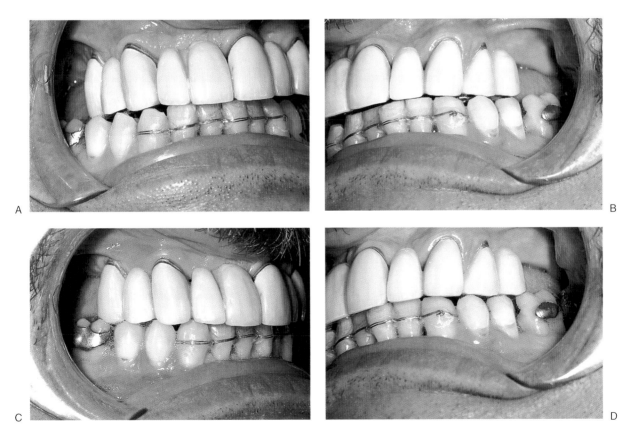

A   B

C   D

Figure 4.10 Restoration to a shortened dental arch after extensive periodontal treatment and the earlier loss of many upper teeth as a result of advanced periodontal disease. (A, B) Ten upper bridge units are supported by five remaining teeth. (C, D) A mutually protected occlusion is achieved; note a bilateral shallow group function with disclusion of the non-working sides.

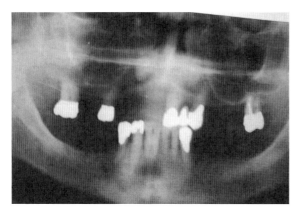

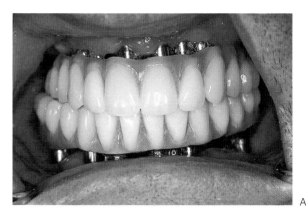

A

Figure 4.11 The pre-treatment radiograph for Patient E, with problems coping with remaining teeth and a partial denture.

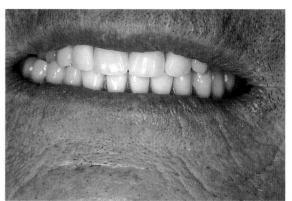

B

upper teeth as a result of advanced periodontal disease. It is essential with a shortened dental arch that all features of a mutually protected occlusion are present (Fig. 4.10C,D).

Full arch implant-supported fixed bridges are usually an example of shortened dental arches. Patient E was 72 years old and was unable to cope with upper and lower partial dentures. The pre-treatment radiograph (Fig. 4.11) shows his remaining teeth, which, though saveable, offered inadequate support for fixed restorations. After elective extraction of most remaining teeth, upper and lower full arch implant-supported bridges were made. The patient then had 12 upper and 11 lower occluding teeth (a shortened arch) but greatly improved function (Fig. 4.12) compared with the initial distribution of teeth supplemented by partial dentures. The upper molars had been retained to support a transitional partial denture, but now their retention is optional. Elective extraction for implant placement is discussed in Chapter 10.

MANAGING TOOTH STRUCTURE LOSS AND VERTICAL DIMENSION

Increasingly, patients present with significant tooth structure loss caused by attrition, erosion or a combination of both. Whereas in the past these patients often progressed to complete dentures, with considerable freedom for the clinician to alter the presenting vertical dimension to achieve aesthetic improvement, they now increasingly hope to retain their remaining teeth. This presents the clinician with a considerable treatment planning challenge. There

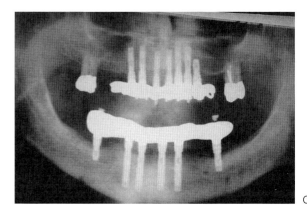

C

Figure 4.12 A full arch implant-supported bridge giving a shortened dental arch for Patient E (A,B). Radiograph shows its placement (C).

are two fundamental questions that the dentist must ask before starting to develop a treatment plan:

- does the patient's vertical dimension need to be altered to achieve the desired result?
- can the patient tolerate the increase in vertical dimension?

Necessity to alter the vertical dimension

The question of changing overall vertical demension can usually be answered by an assessment of the patient's presenting chief complaint combined with a review of mounted study casts. It may well also be necessary to proceed to a diagnostic wax up, both to allow the dentist to assess potential outcomes and to let the patient preview the potential result. If it is possible to achieve an acceptable result without altering vertical dimension, the treatment plan will generally be greatly simplified, since it can usually be carried out in small segments, thus spreading overall costs to the patient as well as giving the dentist an easier task to control the situation.

It is determined that the problems can only be effectively addressed by increasing vertical dimension, both the dentist and the patient are committed to major complex restorative dentistry, which must all be carried out at the same time, since it is clearly not feasible to increase vertical dimension on some teeth but not others.

Patient F, shown in Figure 4.13, is a 45-year-old high school head teacher who wished to improve the appearance of his teeth. Although it may well be technically possible to do so at the present vertical dimension, the smile picture (Fig. 4.13B) shows that insufficient tooth will be visible at this level. To achieve an acceptable result, an increase in vertical dimension to create sufficient space for restorative materials within the aesthetic zone would be necessary.

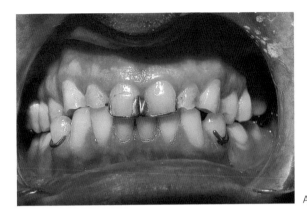

A

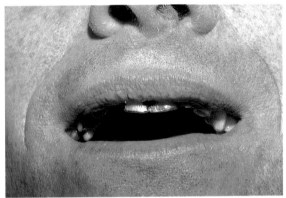

B

Figure 4.13 Patient F: the need to increase vertical dimension. (A) This patient wanted to improve the appearance of his teeth. (B) The smile picture shows that insufficient tooth would be visible at the present vertical dimension.

Can the patient tolerate the increase in vertical dimension?

If it has been determined that an increase in vertical dimension is necessary to achieve restorative objectives, the clinician must now determine if the patient can tolerate this change. Since vertical dimension may have been lost slowly over many years, with a progressive accommodation to the changes, it is never certain that the patient will be able to tolerate the restoration of lost vertical dimension. For this reason, it is mandatory that the increase be tested in a reversible manner before a commitment is made to any form of irreversible treatment. In this way, the patient who cannot tolerate the needed increase can be returned to their presenting condition and be no worse off for the experience.

Patient F (shown before treatment in Fig. 4.13) had the vertical dimension increased by around 4 mm

(Fig. 4.14) by wearing a Hawley bite plane every evening and night. If this can be tolerated, it can provide more than enough space for restorations. Patient F had successfully worn the appliance for 8 weeks, a diagnostic wax-up was made within the new, tested vertical dimension (Fig. 4.15), and temporary crowns were made from this wax up (Fig. 4.16). In order to hold this vertical dimension, acrylic was added to the lower partial denture to establish posterior contact (Fig. 4.17). At this point, it can be confirmed that the patient is happy with the amount of tooth now visible. The upper crown length was increased to improve the retentive length of the preparations (Fig. 4.18). It is necessary to wait at least 16 weeks after this to allow full tissue healing before impressions are taken. The teeth can then be re-prepared (Fig. 4.19) and the upper crowns are taken to completion within the vertical dimension initially tested by the appliance (Fig. 4.20). A modified canine cingulua, which provided centric

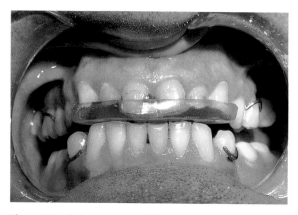

Figure 4.14 Patient tolerance of increased vertical dimension can be assessed by wearing Hawley bite plane every evening and night for 8 weeks at a vertical dimension that will allow adequate space for more cosmetic restorations.

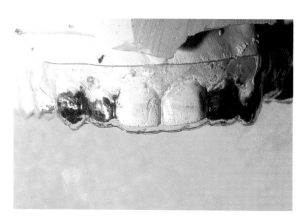

Figure 4.15 A diagnostic wax-up was made for Patient F at the increased vertical dimension and from this a vacuum form stent was formed to allow intraoral fabrication of provisional restorations.

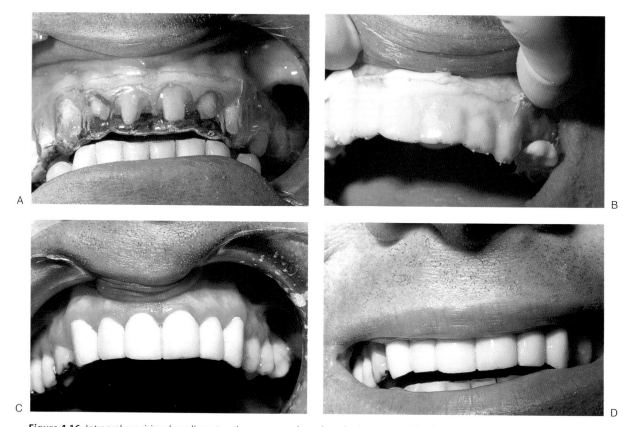

A

B

C

D

Figure 4.16 Intraoral provisional acrylic restorations were made and aesthetics approved by the patient. Compare Figure 4.13.

stops and immediate canine guidance, was incorporated within the crowns (Fig. 4.20C). At a later date, new denture teeth were attached to the satisfactory lower denture framework.

In order to test an increase in vertical dimension in a reversible fashion, the use of an occlusal appliance is widely recommended. There are two schools of thought concerning the approach to increasing

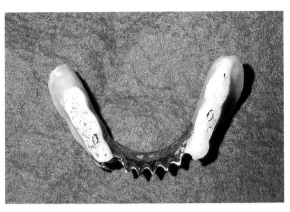
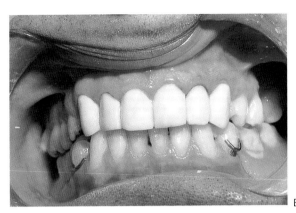

A
B

Figure 4.17 Cold cure acrylic was added to the occlusal surfaces of the lower partial denture to hold the vertical dimension established by the bite plane and upper provisional crowns. Compare Figure 4.13.

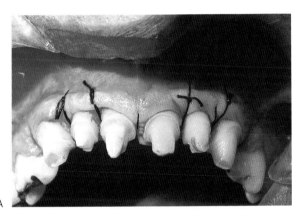
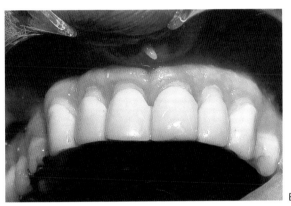

A
B

Figure 4.18 A crown-lengthening procedure was carried out to increase available retentive length for the final crowns for Patient F. It is necessary to wait at least 16 weeks for tissue healing before impressions are taken.

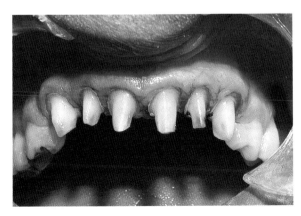

Figure 4.19 After healing, the teeth were re-prepared; note the increase in retentive crown length.

vertical dimension. The first recommends a gradual increment by progressively adding acrylic to a hard splint, around 1 mm per week until the patient reaches the increased vertical needed for restorative purposes. It has been the author's experience that this approach is not only very time consuming but also can lead to an increasingly unhappy patient, who each week has to adapt to a change. The second approach involves taking the patient immediately to the needed increase in vertical dimension or even 1 mm beyond this. Almost all patients tolerate this well; they have to go through considerably less adjustments and the dentist spends much less time. Even in patients who initially experience muscle soreness, a minimal reduction in the vertical dimension of the appliance will generally

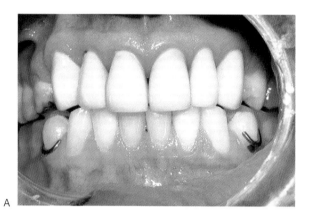

A

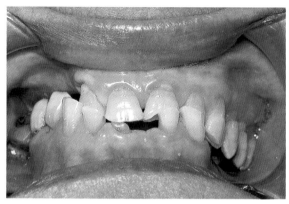

Figure 4.21 Patient G: inability to manage at the presenting vertical dimension. This 64-year-old patient had been advised to have all upper and lower teeth extracted and asked for a second opinion.

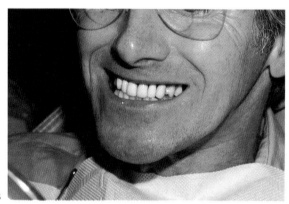

B

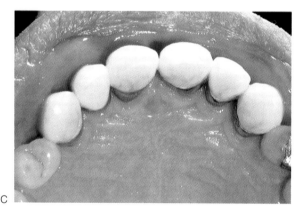

C

Figure 4.20 The restoration for Patient F was completed with the shade and shape of tooth desired by the patient (A, B). A modified canine cingulua was incorporated within the crowns (C) to hold the vertical dimension even when the partial denture was out.

relieve symptoms and establish the range of vertical dimensions within which the restorative dentist can work. Patient G was 64 years of age and had been advised to have all upper and lower teeth extracted. When she presented for a second opinion it was clear

that she could not be managed at the presenting vertical dimension (Fig. 4.21). Because of the need for a major increase of vertical dimension and the problem of distance (the patient travelled over 200 miles for each appointment), it was decided to increase it by over 8 mm in one appointment (Fig. 4.22). This was slightly more than that required for effective restorations. The patient not only tolerated this well, but stated that she had not felt so good for years. Treatment was taken to completion at the new vertical dimension with a combination of fixed and removable prostheses (Fig. 4.23). A night splint was recommended at an even more increased vertical dimension, which was also tolerated well.

To ensure that a patient can tolerate the increase in vertical dimension, it is necessary to have them wear the appliance for at least 12 hours per day (generally evening and night) for a period of 6 to 8 weeks. At this time, if muscles of mastication are flaccid and show no tenderness to palpation, and if temporomandibular joints are free from pain on palpation and opening clicks, then it is usually safe to proceed to more major restorative care.

The patient shown in Figure 4.24 clearly needed an increase in vertical dimension if his severely worn anterior teeth were to be restored. The full cover maxillary splint opened him to a vertical dimension at which aesthetic restorations would be feasible (Fig. 4.24C). After a few weeks, the patient was still complaining of sore muscles with the appliance and, despite reduction in its vertical dimension, eventually stopped wearing it. He decided not to proceed with

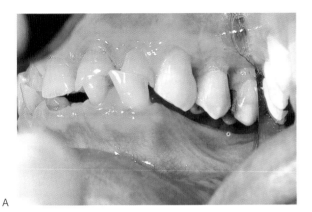

A

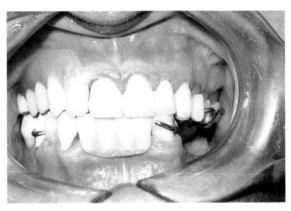

Figure 4.23 Treatment for Patient G was taken to completion at the new vertical dimension with a combination of fixed and removable prostheses. Compare Figure 4.21.

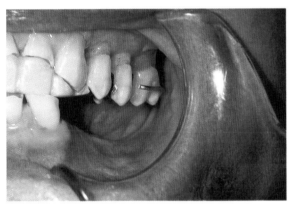

B

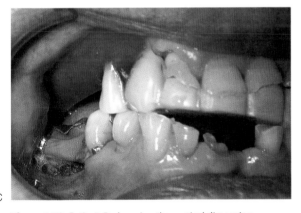

C

Figure 4.22 Patient G: changing the vertical dimension reversibly. An anterior bite plane with tooth-coloured acrylic and two additional teeth on the upper right opened the vertical dimension by over 8 mm.

treatment and, at least, no irreversible treatment had been undertaken. Imaging the problems created if a dentist had proceeded to composites or even crowns at an increased vertical dimension in this patient without first testing the increase in a reversible manner.

Where anterior attrition is severe and several millimetres of opening are needed for restoration of these teeth, the restoration of the posterior occlusion will necessitate an increase in the crown to root ratio of the posterior teeth. The opening will also eliminate any existing anterior guidance, and the overall treatment plan will have to take this into consideration. If it is undesirable to increase posterior crown to root ratios, because of periodontal involvement, short roots or minimally restored teeth, consideration should be given towards achieving a stable posterior occlusion at the desired vertical by intentional posterior eruption. This can be achieved by the use of an anterior bite plane, as has been advocated by Amsterdam, who used a modified Hawley anterior bite plane, and by Dahl, using a chrome cobalt Dahl appliance. It has been the author's experience that the modified Hawley appliance is easier to make and adjust, and it provides considerably more flexibility than the Dahl appliance. For predictable eruption to occur, the appliance should be worn for at least 22 hours per day, and regular monitoring with ongoing occlusal adjustment will be required. If too much opening is incorporated into such an appliance, eruption may be prevented by the development of a lateral tongue thrust.

With any partial coverage appliance there is a risk of undesired eruption, and so when eruption is not intended, partial coverage appliances should only be worn for a maximum of 8 hours per day.

As with all other aspects of treatment, the restoration of teeth that have been subject to tooth structure

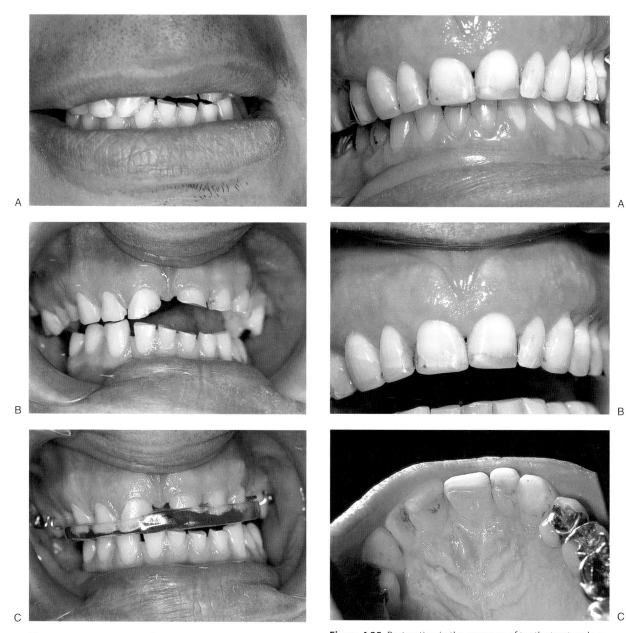

A

B

C

Figure 4.24 A requirement for increased vertical dimension. (A, B) This patient was unhappy with the appearance of his severely worn anterior teeth. (C) A full cover maxillary splint opened the patient to a vertical dimension at which aesthetic restorations would be feasible.

Figure 4.25 Restoration in the presence of tooth structure loss. A mutually protected occlusion has been established with the use of composite resin on upper anterior teeth. In this patient the composites have lasted 5 years to date and can be replaced individually as and when this is required.

loss is best kept as conservative as possible. Where no caries or large past restorations are present, where a mutually protected occlusion can be established, and where sufficient interarch space can be achieved, then composite resin restorations will often provide a good medium-term restoration (Fig. 4.25).

FLEXIBLE PLANNING: ANTICIPATING PROBLEMS AND BUILDING IN SOLUTIONS

It is both presumptuous and unrealistic to expect restorations to last indefinitely. Equally, there are often situations when a tooth adjacent to a new restoration has a doubtful prognosis and may be lost in the foreseeable future. By careful planning with judicious application of Murphy's law 'What's the worst thing that can happen? How could I fix it?' it is often possible to anticipate future problems and build in their possible management without requiring a total remake of the present prosthesis. Situations where this is often feasible include:

- caries under bridge abutments
- potential future loss of a tooth in the arch with a partial denture
- loss of one tooth in a series of crowns
- loss of doubtful tooth that is a key bridge abutment
- loss of a doubtful tooth adjacent to an implant-supported prosthesis
- fracture of a filling or cusp under a new partial denture
- longer term use of temporary cementation.

Caries under a bridge abutment

Figure 4.26 shows caries that has developed under two abutments of a 6-unit bridge, which had been satisfactory for 9 years. The patient (at age 75) would prefer not to have a new bridge. Since the bridge was successfully removed in one piece, it was feasible to salvage the present bridge. Endodontics was completed on 1-3 and 1-1 and all caries was removed, completely clearing the remaining tooth structure from the bridge (Fig. 4.27). Individual post and core impressions (Fig. 4.28A) were taken (other types of material could be used). A locating Durelay impression

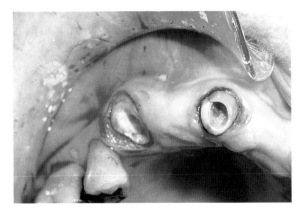

Figure 4.27 The bridge was successfully removed in one piece. Endodontics was completed on teeth 1-3 and 1-1 and all caries was removed, completely clearing the remaining tooth structure from the bridge.

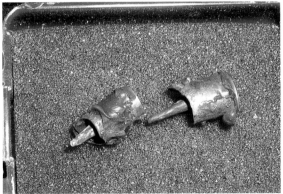

A

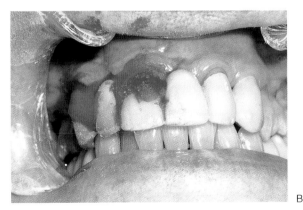

B

Figure 4.28 Bridge repair. (A) Individual copper band and compound impressions for post, core and collars were taken. (B) A locating Durelay impression was taken to locate the dies in relation to the bridge.

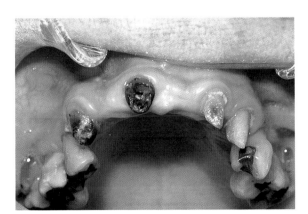

Figure 4.26 Restoration for caries under a bridge abutment. Caries has developed under two abutments of a 6-unit bridge.

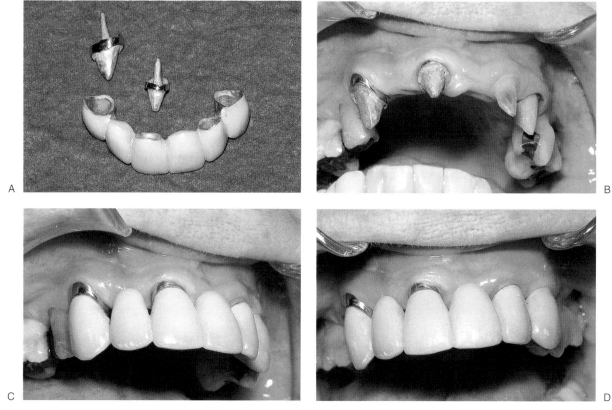

A

B

C

D

Figure 4.29 (A–C) Cast metal post, core and collars were made, cemented and the bridge was re-cemented. (D) The repaired bridge lasted for the remaining 6 years of the patient's life.

within the bridge was taken (Fig. 4.28B) by painting the Durelay into the preparations and the entrance to the root canals, thus filling the fitting surface of the bridge with Durelay and seating it. The patient closed into the intercuspal position to ensure full seating. This will allow location of the dies from the copper band impressions in relation to the bridge. Cast metal post, core and collars were made, cemented and the bridge was re-cemented (Fig. 4.29A–C). The bridge lasted for the remaining 6 years of the patient's life (Fig. 4.29D).

Potential future loss of a tooth in the same arch as a new partial denture

Where one of the remaining teeth supporting a partial denture has a doubtful prognosis, the denture framework should be designed for easy addition of the doubtful tooth. The partial denture in Figure 4.30 was designed with a lingual mesh to allow the simple addition of one or more of the remaining incisors should they be lost.

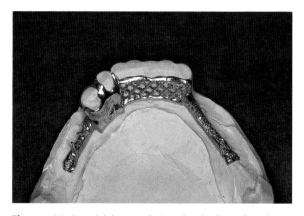

Figure 4.30 A partial denture designed with a lingual mesh to allow the simple addition of one or more of the remaining incisors should they be lost.

Loss of one tooth in a series of crowns

Judicious 'preventive' splinting can often offer a simple solution to an otherwise major problem. The patient in Figure 4.31 had had three lower (and 10 upper)

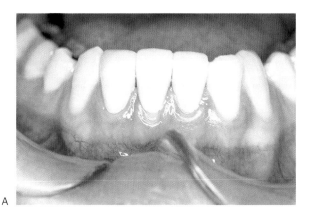

A

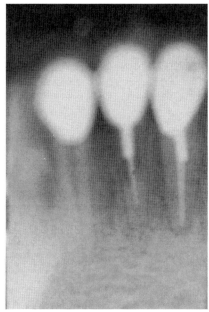

B

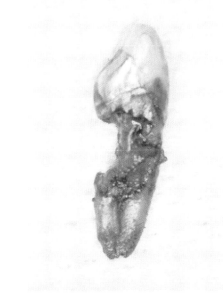

A

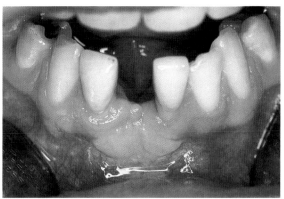

B

Figure 4.31 Loss of one of a series of crowns. (A) Three lower crowns placed after trauma when several teeth had been loosened and displaced. (B) Within 2 years of crown placement, extensive internal root resorption occurred on tooth 4-1.

Figure 4.32 The tooth failing in Figure 4.31 was extracted with great care (A), preserving as much bone as possible. (B) After healing the patient required either a single implant or a new 3-unit bridge, with removal of two perfectly good crowns.

crowns placed after trauma in a major automobile accident. Her history indicated that several teeth were loosened and displaced in the accident. Within 2 years of crown placement, extensive internal root resorption had occurred on tooth 4-1 (Figure 4.31B). The tooth was extracted preserving as much bone as possible (Figure 4.32A) but the patient then required either a single implant or a new 3-unit bridge and removal of two perfectly good crowns (Fig. 4.32B). Where the prognosis of any of the teeth to be crowned is doubtful, as in this case, judicious splinting of the crowns would have negated the need for total re-treatment.

There is a risk of up to 15% of a root canal-treated tooth with a post and core developing a later vertical root fracture. Patient H, Figure 4.33, was a young dental hygiene student who had four large post and cores supporting crowns on her upper incisors, which had been traumatised when she was a child. The crowns were unaesthetic and had poor marginal fit. They required replacement after cosmetic periodontal surgery. Because of the high risk of future root fracture on at least one of the teeth, it was decided to splint the crowns together (Fig. 4.34) so that such a problem can be managed.

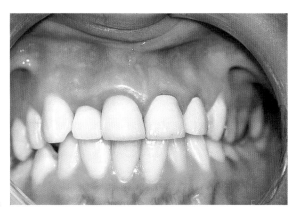
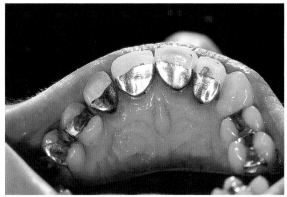

A   B

Figure 4.33 Preventive splinting. Four crowns in Patient H were unaesthetic, had poor marginal fit and required replacement.

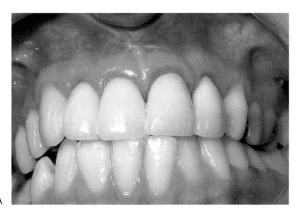
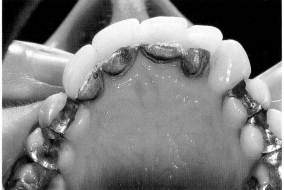

A   B

Figure 4.34 Patient H: preventive splinting. The replacement crowns were splinted because of the high risk of root fracture in such teeth.

Four years later, Patient H re-presented with a vertical root fracture on tooth 1-2 (Fig. 4.35). With a conservative flap procedure the root was carefully removed (Fig. 4.36A), the socket filled with hydro-xyapatite crystals (Fig. 4.36B) and covered with a Gore Tex membrane (Fig. 4.36C) and sutured closed (Fig. 4.36D). Ten weeks later at the time of Gore Tex removal, good early bone regeneration was occurring (Fig. 4.37). The patient maintained good cosmetics, with the original splinted crowns converted to a cantilever bridge (Fig. 4.38). In this way 'preventive' splinting allowed the extension of the life of these crowns. All that was necessary was a knowledge of risks, care to prepare the teeth parallel to each other, and a flexible approach to treatment planning for the long term.

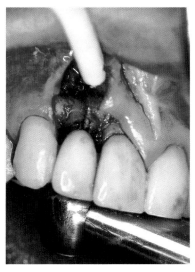

Figure 4.35 A vertical root fracture on tooth 1-2 in Patient H, 4 years after replacement crowns.

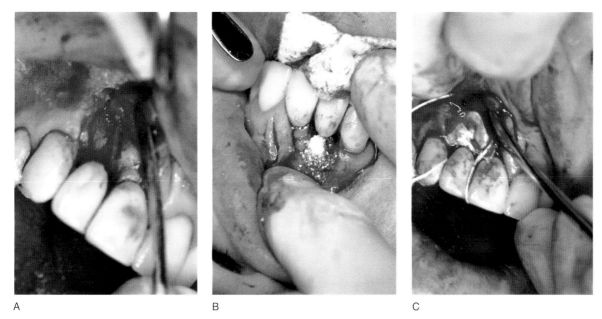

A   B   C

Figure 4.36 Patient H: management of the vertical root fracture. (A) With a conservative flap procedure the root was carefully removed. (B) The socket was filled with hydroxyapatite crystals. (C) The graft material was covered with a Gore Tex regenerative membrane. (D) The extraction site was carefully sutured closed.

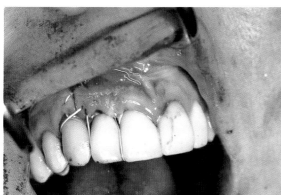

D

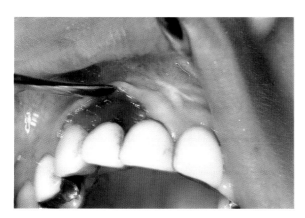

Figure 4.37 Good early bone regeneration was occurring when the Gore Tex membrane was removed 10 weeks later.

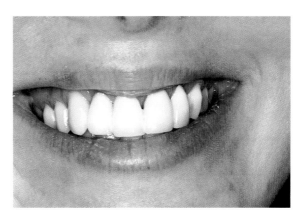

Figure 4.38 The use of 'preventive splinting' in Patient H, which anticipated possible future problems, enabled good cosmetics to be preserved with the original splinted crowns, now converted to a cantilever bridge.

Loss of a doubtful tooth, that is a key bridge abutment

Where a key bridge abutment has a doubtful long-term prognosis, the bridge should be designed for possible future extension. This is achieved by having the laboratory place a flat metal contact point distal to the terminal abutment and cementing the bridge with a temporary cement. If and when the abutment fails, the tooth or teeth distal to the bridge can be prepared as additional abutments, and the new abutments post-soldered to the original bridge. Figure 4.39 shows a vertical root fracture on tooth 2-3 in Patient I. This was the key abutment on a 10-unit bridge from 1-5 to 2-5, replacing all incisors as well as the right canine. Because Patient I gave a history of root fractures and presented originally with a large post in tooth 2-3, this potential problem had been anticipated when the bridge was made 3 years previously. Two years later, the patient re-presented with a subgingival fracture of 2-3. The upper molars distal to the bridge were prepared parallel to the bridge abutments (Fig. 4.40) and then indexed in Durelay to relate them to the original bridge (Fig. 4.40B). The sections were then post-soldered (Fig. 4.40C,D). The split root was then carefully extracted (Fig. 4.41A,B), the hollow area under 2-3 filled with composite and customised to the socket (Fig. 4.41C), and the extended bridge (now 14 units) re-cemented (Fig. 4.41D). This extended bridge has served the patient for an additional 12 years to date. The only additional effort required to ensure this ability to salvage a problem situation is to take a few more moments in the writing of the laboratory prescription, and in the use of temporary cement.

Loss of a doubtful tooth adjacent to an implant-supported prosthesis

It is often the situation that an implant-supported prosthesis is made adjacent to a tooth with a doubtful prognosis. While ideally this tooth might be extracted and incorporated in the original prosthesis, the patient will on occasion not allow this. In such cases, the implant-supported prosthesis should be designed to allow possible future addition. Patient J presented with no teeth behind the upper first premolar (tooth 1-4), which had an incomplete root canal filling and limited remaining tooth structure (Fig. 4.42). Although advised that this tooth may best be extracted and incorporated in an implant supported bridge, she declined and agreed on a compromise plan of retaining the tooth and placing two implants to replace 1-5 and 1-6 (Fig. 4.43). Custom abutments were made (Fig. 4.43B). It was decided that the splinted implant-supported crowns would incorporate a flat metal mesial contact point on 1-5 to allow for future addition of 1-4 if it were ever lost (Fig. 4.43C,D). Two years later, 1-4 fractured well subgingivally (Fig. 4.44) and Patient J agreed to extraction. An immediate 3-unit provisional bridge was made (Fig. 4.45) and this was inserted at the time of extraction (Fig. 4.45B). After socket healing was complete, a pick-up impression of the original bridge was made and a pontic post-soldered in the laboratory (Fig. 4.46). This extended prosthesis was then recemented (Fig. 4.47). Again only few more moments in the writing of the laboratory prescription, and the use of temporary cement were necessary to first anticipate and then salvage this situation.

Fracture of a filling or cusp under a new partial denture

When a new metal partial denture is being constructed, a careful assessment should be made of all teeth that will support its framework. Not only should the partial denture design accommodate possible loss of teeth with doubtful prognosis (see Fig. 4.30), but also the individual restorations on each abutment tooth should be critically appraised for potential future

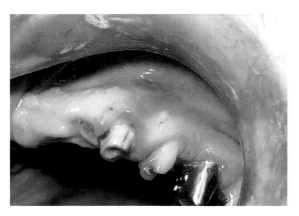

Figure 4.39 Patient I: anticipating future loss of a key abutment. A vertical root fracture has developed on tooth 2-3, which is a key abutment on a 10-unit bridge that had been designed for possible addition of more distal abutments if a problem arose.

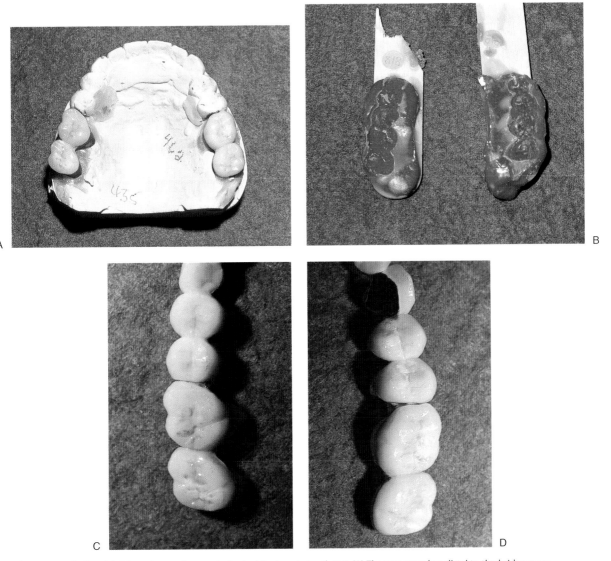

Figure 4.40 Patient I: bridge salvage after a subgingival fracture in tooth 2-3. (A) The upper molars distal to the bridge were prepared parallel to the bridge abutments, splinted crowns tried in at the bisque bake for occlusal refinement, then glazed. The first molars had flat mesial contact points. (B) These new crowns were indexed in the mouth with Durelay to relate them to the original bridge. (C, D) After drying out the original bridge for a few hours, the sections were post-soldered, converting the prosthesis to 14 units.

problems. The patient in Figure 4.48 had recently had a new partial denture constructed. Within 6 months, the buccal cusp of the upper second premolar, which already had an MOD (mesio-occluso-distal) amalgam, had fractured. Close inspection showed that the cast metal clasp engaged the tooth just opposite the floor of the amalgam, just where the cusp is likely to be weakest. The clinician then was faced with the choice

of attempting to place a larger filling or a crown under the existing partial denture, and any dentist who has attempted this knows how difficult it can be, or making a new partial denture once a new restoration has been placed. Either way the dentist is faced with the dilemma of either having to adsorb costs to preserve good will or having a problem patient if billed for another partial denture within 6 months of the

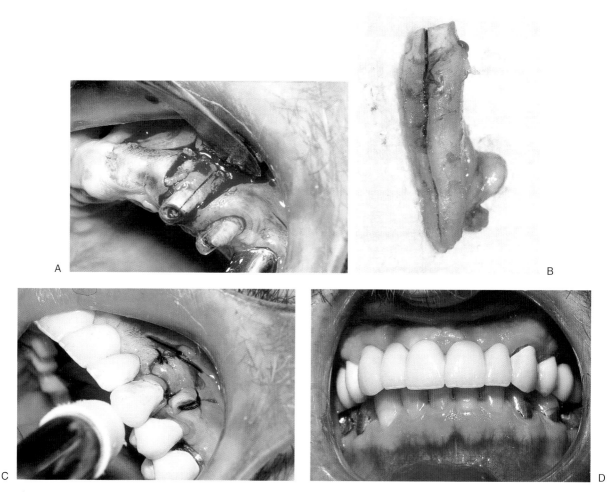

A
B
C
D

Figure 4.41 Patient I: removal of the split root. (A, B) Using a conservative flap approach, the split root was carefully extracted. (C) The underside of crown 2-3 was sandblasted, filled with composite and customised to the socket. (D) The bridge was re-cemented and continued to serve Patient I for many more years.

first. Such situations can usually be prevented by advising replacement of doubtful restorations on abutment teeth. If the patient declines and is advised of the possible consequences, than a dentist can feel much more comfortable about charging for a remake when such a complication arises.

Longer term use of temporary cementation

Dentists must put themselves in the patient's place when considering offering to 'patch' a defect on a relatively new restoration. Few of us would accept a plastic patch on a hole that appears on the bodywork of a relatively new car. How then can we expect a patient to accept a composite or amalgam filling over an access preparation when a root canal problem

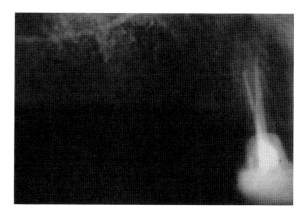

Figure 4.42 Patient J: an implant-supported restoration adjacent to a doubtful tooth. Implant replacement of teeth 1-5 and 1-6 was adjacent to tooth 1-4, which had a poor root canal filling and limited remaining tooth structure.

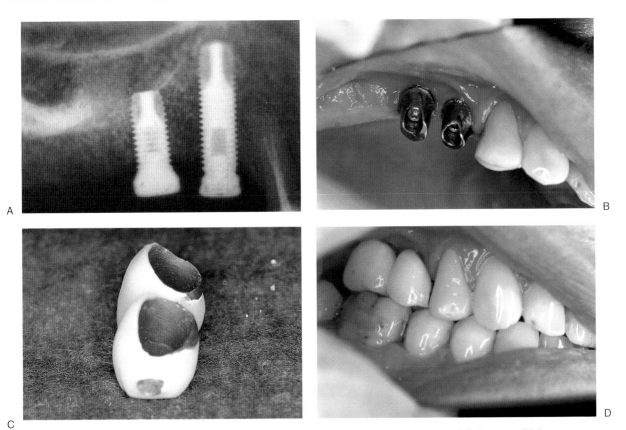

Figure 4.43 Implant crowns to allow for future additions. (A) Two implants were placed and successfully integrate. (B) Custom abutments were made to support the implant prosthesis. (C, D) The implant crowns were designed with a flat metal mesial contact point on 1-5 to allow for future addition of 1-4 if it is ever lost.

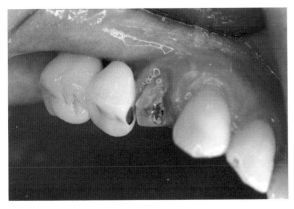

Figure 4.44 Patient J: 2 years later, tooth 1-4 fractured subgingivally and was unrestorable. Note the metal mesial contact on 2-5.

has developed under a new crown? We know that around 20 to 25% all teeth prepared for crowns will subsequently need root canal fillings, and so surely we should anticipate this and plan for the eventuality. The judicious use of long-term temporary cementation can provide adequate retention, while allowing retrievability when needed. Endodontics carried out after a crown is removed is much more conservative of tooth structure, maintains better retention for the restoration once it has been recemented, and avoids cutting through the occlusal of the crown.

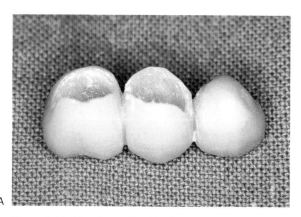

A

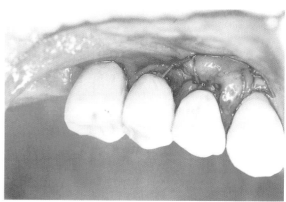

B

Figure 4.45 A 3-unit provisional bridge was made to be supported by the two implants (see Fig. 4.43). The provisional bridge (A) was inserted in conjunction with the extraction of tooth 1-4 (B).

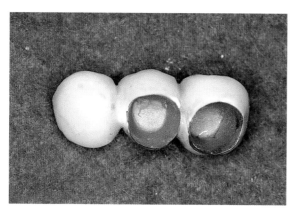

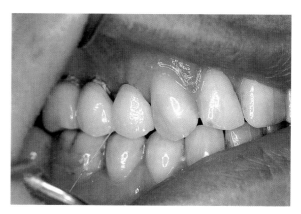

Figure 4.46 After socket healing a porcelain bonded to gold alloy pontic was made and post-soldered to the original splinted implant crowns.

Figure 4.47 The modified prosthesis was re-cemented and continued to serve Patient J.

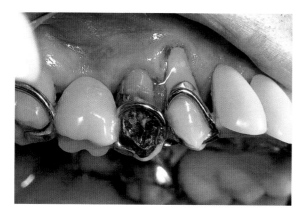

Figure 4.48 Fracture of a buccal cusp of the upper second premolar within 6 months of constructing a new partial denture.

5 Case presentation: communicating with the patient

ORGANISATION PRIOR TO CASE PRESENTATION

While it is often feasible, in simple cases, to present treatment options to a patient at the same visit as data gathering, there are many situations where it is necessary to review data, study models and radiographs, and even consult with colleagues, before developing treatment options and presenting these. The dentist should not rush, or be rushed, into developing instant treatment plans in complex situations. Although dentists do not like to be compared with various tradesmen, we would probably expect an immediate quote for repair of a broken window but would be suspicious of an instant estimate for an extension to our home. In more complex cases, we should be prepared to bring the patient back for a separate case presentation appointment. If there is a significant delay before this can be booked, then it is often wise to send the patient a letter outlining the treatment options that have been developed and to use the presentation visit to review the recommendations, answer any questions arising and hopefully reach an agreement on the treatment plan to be followed.

It must be accepted that most patients are not qualified to judge the diagnostic and clinical skill of their general dentist. Criteria such as 'not hurting', 'fillings and crowns not falling out', 'being nice and being fairly cheap' are more likely to be used than how well caries is removed, the efficiency of root planning or the density of a gutta percha root filling.

While we realise that there is a vast range of skills, knowledge and interest within the dental profession—D. Walter Cohen (Dean Emeritus, University of Pennsylvania School of Dental Medicine) said: 'Never forget that half of the dentists graduated in the bottom half of their class'—many patients assume that all dentists are more or less the same and judge them using incomplete, subjective criteria. For this reason, we must be sensitive to the manner and environment in which we present treatment options to our patients. In essence, we must try to make a good first impression, conveying an air of preparedness, competence, thoroughness and empathy, which will hopefully differentiate our 'product' from that of our 'competitors'.

There are certain basics that should be observed in order to convey the appropriate impression:

- X-ray films should be mounted and clearly have the patient's name on them
- study models should be well trimmed, and, when mounted, the articulator should be clean (Fig. 5.1A).
- any correspondence should be printed and well laid out
- the dentist should have a clear idea of the treatment options to be presented and the order in which these are to be discussed
- examples of similar cases, be they in book, model or computer graphic form should be readily to hand
- informational brochures should be to hand
- the environment for presentation, either in the operatory or a separate room, should be clean, uncluttered and comfortable (Fig. 5.1B). It is important to get the patient out of the dental chair to allow them to relax a bit, knowing that, at least for now, the threat of potential discomfort (other than financial) is past.

THE CASE PRESENTATION ENVIRONMENT

Location

It is ideal if a case presentation can take place outwith the treatment area (Fig. 5.1B). Apart from the clear benefit of using a custom-made, more relaxed environment, it also provides the opportunity for another staff member to prepare and possibly even use the treatment area for another patient. While this separate area is often considered a luxury and a non-revenue-generating area, it may more than pay for itself both in a higher level of patient acceptance for advanced

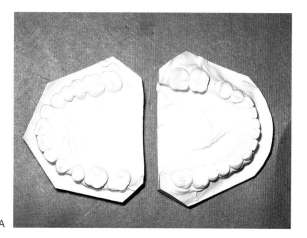

A

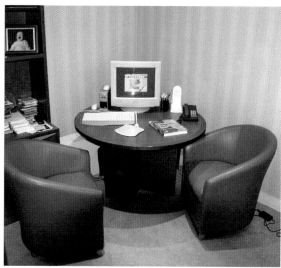

B

Figure 5.1 Giving the patient the right impression. (A) Well-trimmed tidy study models will convey an impression of preparedness and organisation to the patient. (B) A clean, uncluttered comfortable presentation area.

treatment and by freeing the treatment area for additional treatment to be carried out. Clearly the size and layout of the practice will influence the practicality of having such an area. Care should be taken to create a relaxed atmosphere of comfort rather than luxury. It is human nature for many patients to wonder if quoted fees are justified, and while family photographs and pleasing décor convey a positive impression, Picassos and photographs of the dentist's yacht are likely to prompt a negative reaction. A few well-selected framed professional certificates may be beneficial, but a wall of flimsy certificates that are essentially receipts for attending meetings are generally seen through by most patients.

Where it is impractical to have a separate room, and the treatment area is to be used, the dentist should try to get the patient out of the dental chair and, at the least, seat them on an assistant's stool or a normal chair so that both dentist and patient are sitting at the same level, either at a table or work surface. By using this type of arrangement, the dentist's body language conveys the message 'lets work out together how to fix these problems' rather than the 'here's how I'm going to fix your teeth' message that is conveyed by the dentist talking down to a patient who is still in the dental chair. This table surface should be uncluttered and with enough space to accommodate a radiograph viewer, models, computer terminal if used and relevant paperwork. The patient and dentist should, as far as possible, be in equivalent positions and chairs.

Visual aids

Digital intraoral cameras and computer technology

With major advances in digital intraoral cameras and computer technology, it is feasible to show the patient in real time close-up pictures of their mouth and to explain their problems in ways not previously possible. While these are invaluable tools in a case presentation, the dentist should take care not to get too involved in the technology rather than the patient and should focus primarily on the solutions rather than the problems. Computer graphics are sufficiently advanced to allow us to carry out sophisticated 'virtual dentistry' on the computer screen in an apparently painless, bloodless and instantaneous manner. Real dentistry is not so simple, and care must be taken to avoid selling something that cannot be delivered. Polaroid pictures, especially taken at varying angles (Fig. 5.2), can be useful where an intraoral camera is not available. Sparingly used, intraoral pictures will be effective in assisting in a case presentation.

Younger dentists must be aware of the resistance to some technological advances by 'baby boomers' and older patients. Most research suggests that the average age of patients who agree to (and can afford) advanced care such as implants or major bridgework is between 50 and 60 years. The skilled dentist should be able to customise the format of a presentation to the age and attitude of the patient.

The hand mirror

For several generations, dentists and hygienists have used hand mirrors both to show the patient problems

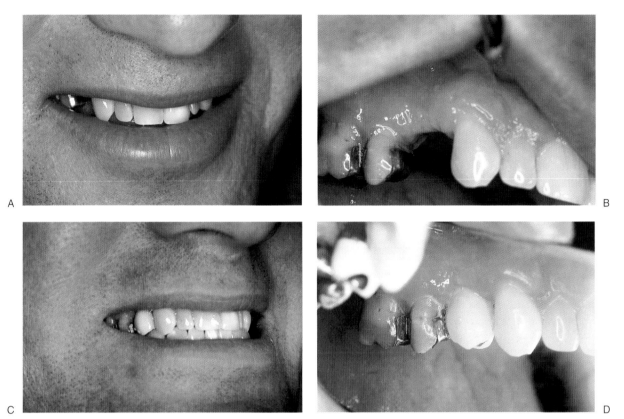

A

B

C

D

Figure 5.2 The use of photographs to convey information. (A) This patient could not understand why his wife complained about the space in the upper right premolar region. When he looked at himself in the mirror, the space was not evident. (B) However, when shown a photograph from just around 20% to the right he became aware of the space and decided to proceed with treatment. (C, D) The missing tooth was replaced by an implant-supported crown and the patient and his wife are happy.

in their own mouth and to instruct them in oral hygiene. Older patients may prefer this more familiar technology; it also allows an initial 'in mouth' approach before going to a table-top or computer screen presentation and so establishes a chain of relevance to the latter. It can also be useful to stand behind a patient as they look in a mirror to see what they see, and importantly to see what is missed with the straight-on anterior view. Often a missing upper premolar is not evident in the front mirror view; however, when the patient is shown an angled photograph to allow them to see themselves as others see them, they can be motivated towards tooth replacement (Fig. 5.2 A,B).

Radiographs

In addition to their diagnostic value, radiographs can be invaluable visual aid in case presentation. They can easily illustrate the presence of an overhanging margin,

caries under a restoration, apical areas and particularly bone loss. By illustrating what cannot be easily seen clinically, they compliment the camera or mirror. The dentist must not assume that a patient understands what they see and must take care to explain the simple landmarks: the white of metal restorations and root fillings, the normal and present position of bone and other important structures such as the maxillary sinus and inferior dental canal. It is often beneficial to make a simple drawing of the key features on the radiographs so that these can be labelled and alternative treatment options illustrated.

Study casts and diagnostic wax ups

Again casts and wax ups can compliment the other aids outlined above. They are particularly useful in illustrating overeruption and tipping of teeth, as well as allowing the patient to see the extent of crowding or spacing. By using models to develop a diagnostic wax up of a possible restorative or orthodontic correction, the clinician can both assess the feasibility of these approaches and use the models to allow the patient to visualise the final result. Diagnostic wax ups have the advantage over computer simulations of being truly three-dimensional in nature, and of allowing the patient to actually hold the models and, if desired, take them home to discuss with other family members. In complex cases, it may well be necessary to carry out an initial presentation with regular study models presenting tentative treatment options, and then have the patient return for a supplementary presentation if they express an interest in one of the more advanced options.

Laboratory-produced models with restorative examples

In the author's experience laboratory-produced models are of only limited value. Such models are invariably expensive, not easily updated as new treatment options come along and tend to be cluttered by the laboratory trying to incorporate several types of restoration on one set of models. They can confuse the patient by often incorporating options that are not applicable. Their main use is often in educating a new member of staff in what is involved in various procedures offered in the practice.

Books and brochures

Many companies now produce both individual brochures illustrating specific treatments for various situations and larger volumes of various treatment options with abundant illustrations. While these are extremely useful in educating patients, they have the limitation of being someone-else's work and, with brochures, are often slanted towards one treatment approach. Hence a brochure on single tooth replacement produced by an implant company is unlikely to present full coverage and resin-retained bridges in the most favourable light. Since the 1980s, Goldstein's 'Changing your smile' has proved to be an invaluable waiting room coffee table book.

Scrapbook and websites showing completed cases

Both scrapbooks and websites are time consuming to develop but they have the benefits of both showing cases treated within the dentist's practice and being easy to edit and update. Again care should be taken in ensuring a high-quality professional presentation, and in avoiding too many pictures per case. Befores and afters are best; surgical pictures are best avoided and happy smiling patients are invaluable. Ambiguous information such as visible metal margins when lips are retracted should either be avoided or complimented with a smile picture with the lips in place showing the patient what is seen by the outside world. Examples can be seen at www.edinburghdentist.com It is often beneficial to refer the patient to the website even before the initial consultation since this allows them to browse in their own time.

VERBAL COMMUNICATIONS WITH THE PATIENT

Although the written word can and should be used to outline and clarify all complex treatment proposals and estimates of fees, it is the dentist's verbal communication that will have the most impact on the patient's final decision on treatment. Both what is said and how it is said is important in developing the level of comfort within the patient that will encourage their acceptance of treatment proposals. In terms of what to say or not say, it is essential to avoid use of emotive words and to use non-emotive equivalents. Hence, 'I plan to give you an injection at the back of your mouth, peel back your gums, grind any uneven bone, scrape your roots and then stitch your gums back' is less likely to elicit a positive response than 'I would like your permission to carefully numb the area, gently ease back the tissue and, after cleaning your root surfaces and repairing any hard tissue damage, I will reposition the gums carefully back in place'. Both describe the same procedure and yet the latter sounds significantly more bearable than the former. Examples of emotive words and their non-emotive equivalents are given in Table 5.1. The reader should also note the use of modifying adverbs such as *gently* and *carefully* to reduce the potential emotion attached to a procedure and to imprint the image of a gentle caring practitioner.

The verbal presentation should stress the health and quality of life gains of proposed treatment rather than attempt to justify the proposed fees with details of the complexity of procedures or length of appointment time involved. Hence phrases such as 'Look better', 'feel better', 'last longer', 'allow you to chose any foods from the menu' and 'give you more confidence' should be used rather than going into details of material

Table 5.1 Emotive and non-emotive equivalent terms

Emotive	Non-emotive equivalent
Drill	Remove, shape
Cut	Shape, separate, remove
Needle	Numb
Pain	Discomfort
This won't hurt	You may feel a little, brief discomfort
Bleeding	Oozing
Swelling	Puffiness

strength, laboratory stages or consequences of not following recommendations.

The verbal presentation can be used in advance of a letter outlining treatment options or can be used to review and answer questions after a letter has been sent. In the most complex cases, this follow-up discussion can help to bring the patient to a final decision and ensure informed consent before treatment commences. To avoid the impression of a hard sell it is useful to use phrases such as:

- I think that is the best advise I can give you
- Are you quite comfortable with that?
- I feel that these are all reasonable options.

It is important to avoid using dental jargon whenever possible. Although some patients will be able to work out where **occluso-buccal** is, it is better to talk about the *front* and *outside* of the tooth. A **composite filling** should be described as a *white filling* and the **periodontium** is better described as the *gums and other tissues that hold the teeth*. Every dentist will have his/her own style of presenting options to a patient, and overall it is better to avoid making too many significant changes, which may sound artificial.

Also within the realm of verbal communications is the option of putting the patient in touch with another patient who has had a similar procedure. The author has found this particularly beneficial in areas of dentistry where patients may not have direct or family experience. Many patients who have had implants or adult orthodontics are willing, and indeed enthusiastic, about discussing treatment with prospective patients. By stressing that you must get the previous patient's permission first, the dentist is also reinforcing the respect for confidentiality within your practice.

WRITTEN COMMUNICATIONS WITH PATIENT

Ultimately the written communication with the patient will constitute the formal basis on which complex treatment is proposed and accepted or rejected. As well as clarifying and reviewing findings and treatment proposals (Fig. 5.3), already discussed with the patient, it will generally incorporate an estimate of fees (Fig. 5.4), clarify payment arrangements or options and, from the medico-legal perspective, enter the patient's records to document what has been advised. Some legal systems require a signed agreement to the treatment proposals, while others accept commencement of proposed treatment as implied consent to the terms and conditions of the treatment plan. This is discussed in detail in Chapter 9.

When the treatment plan options have been developed using a problem list, it is useful to incorporate the active problems, in lay terms, into the letter (Fig. 5.3). Obviously simple treatment plans will not require complex letters and a patient needing a couple of fillings and a scaling and polishing is generally well managed with purely verbal information. However, since most practice management software packages incorporate the facility to generate a written estimate at the front desk with little effort, it is good practice to provide this in all but the simplest treatment plans. If a plumber, carpenter or electrician is prepared to take the time to provide a written estimate, surely a dental professional should be prepared to do the same.

DISCUSSING FEES

Anyone who provides a service for a fee should be prepared to discuss these fees with the potential client or patient. The dentist is in the best position to answer a patient's questions on fees, and even the best-trained auxiliary is unlikely to have sufficient training and experience to field some questions. Most dentists are uncomfortable discussing fees with patients. This is largely a consequence of a failure in dental education to train the dentist for this task, as well as an insecurity on the part of some dentists to propose fees that they, themselves, may hesitate over if in the patient's position.

It is the author's opinion that in most situations the dentist, and not an auxiliary, should raise the question of fees. It is simple to lead into this discussion with a phrase such as 'You are probably wondering about the costs involved in these treatment options'. Of course

Dentist's name
Dentist's qualifications
Any specialist qualification

Dentist's surgery address
Telephone, Fax and emergency numbers

Mr A. Patient   Date
86 Some Road
Anytown

Dear Mr Patient,

It was a pleasure to meet you earlier this month and I am writing, as promised, to outline my findings and recommendations. As I explained, I found you to have the following problems and considerations, which should be addressed as part of your dental treatment.

- A failing bridge on your upper front teeth, which is very mobile and only supported by one tooth. I feel that this tooth (tooth 1-1) has a very poor future. The other tooth no longer supports the bridge due to cement failure. While it has a good bone support, it may have nerve damage.
- A fractured upper right molar (tooth 1-6) which has a very poor future.
- An upper right molar (tooth 1-7) with a crown missing. This tooth is very tapered and has poor retention for a crown.
- A temporary filling on your upper left canine tooth, where you had recent pain. This tooth will likely need root canal treatment.
- An abscess under the tooth in front of the space on your lower left (tooth 3-5).
- Decay, on your lower right, under the old crown (on tooth 4-5) and under an old filling (tooth 4-4).
- Open margins under two crowns on your upper left. These are at high risk of decay.
- Overcontoured, excessively bulky crowns on your lower molars. While these are presently sound, they may cause an unecessary build up of plaque and increase the risk of decay and gum disease,
- Areas of ineffective homecare, allowing plaque build up.
- Your desire to avoid a partial denture, at least in the long-run.

I feel that we should accept the loss of two teeth (teeth 1-6 and 1-1) and focus on retaining the rest and the overall management of your dental problems. Based on my findings and your wishes, I would advise the following treatment plan to manage these problems. This is best divided into phases.

Active Disease Control

1. Fabrication of mounted study models to finalise treatment planning.
2. Preparation of a temporary immediate partial denture replacing upper central incisors.
3. Removal of your upper front bridge and careful extraction of teeth 1-6 and 1-1.
4. Likely placement of a bone graft and/or bone regenerative membrane into the sockets to preserve bone for possible future implant placement.
5. Raising of tissue around tooth 1-7 to improve future crown support.
6. Insertion of temporary immediate partial denture with possible reline.
7. Modification of present crown or fabrication of a temporary crown on tooth 2-2.

Figure 5.3 An example of a letter reviewing findings and treatment proposals.

8. Removal of present restorations on teeth 4-4 and 4-5 and likely root canal treatment on these teeth. These teeth may be found to be too far gone to be restorable in the future.
9. Completion of root canal treatment on teeth 2-3, 3-5 and possibly 1-2, 4-4 and 4-5.
10. Final filling on tooth 2-3.
11. Full mouth scaling and polishing with review of oral hygiene methods.
12. Reassessment. At this point we would have stabilised active disease and would know the prognosis of teeth 4-4 and 4-5. We would then finalise the advanced restorative phase of your treatment. While I can outline this in general terms at present, details can only be finalised once active disease has been controlled and oral hygiene improved.

Advanced Restorative Care (tentative plan)

1. Possible additional periodontal surgery to increase the retention on teeth to support crowns and bridges.
2. Four- to six-tooth upper front bridge replacing upper central incisors or two implant supported crowns replacing upper central incisors and a single crown on tooth 1-2.
3. Cast metal posts and cores on some or all of root canal-treated teeth, which are having crowns or bridges.
4. A three-toothed bridge on your upper right.
5. A three-toothed bridge on your lower left.
6. Crowns on teeth 4-4 and 4-5 if these can be saved.
7. Replacement of crowns on your upper left and lower right. While these should ideally be replaced soon, this could be delayed for a year or two unless active decay started.
8. Fabrication of a night-time appliance to protect the new restorations.

Maintenance Phase

You should be prepared to carry out good daily homecare, have 1 hour with an experienced dental hygienist every 3 months and have annual comprehensive examinations.

If you wished, the advance restorative phase could be carried out in stages, with replacement of the upper front teeth taking first priority. If this approach was taken, you may need a series of night-time appliances as work progresses.

If all goes well I would expect this treatment to take between 9 and 14 months to complete. You should be aware that implant success rates on the upper jaw are around 90% in non-smokers. In the event of an implant failing, it is generally possible to replace it within a few months. This would, however, inevitably extend treatment time. In addition to the possibility of implant failure, there is also around a 20% risk of a few days' swelling and/or bruising, and a slight risk (less than 1%) of damage to the nerve of an adjacent tooth, leading to the need for root canal treatment. Percentage success rates are provided to allow you to reach an informed decision on treatment. There can be absolutely no guarantee that any implant will succeed in an individual case. I would stress that long-term success is also dependent on continued good oral hygiene, regular professional cleanings and monitoring as advised. I have enclosed an estimate for the parts of your treatment that I can provide.

I realise that these are complex treatment proposals and that you may have some questions. Please feel free to call at any time. If you wish to proceed with treatment, please call Angela at the number above and she will coordinate your care.

Yours sincerely,

Dentist's name

Figure 5.3, cont'd

ESTIMATE OF FEES

Mr A. Patient

Active Disease Control

1.	Fabrication of mounted study models to finalise treatment planning	£ 90
2.	Preparation of a temporary immediate partial denture.	230
3.	Removal of your upper front bridge; careful extraction of 1-6 and 1-1	290
4.	Bone graft and/or bone regenerative membrane	300
5.	Raising of tissue around tooth 1-7 to improve future crown support	150
6.	Insertion of temporary immediate partial denture with possible reline	40
7.	Modification or fabrication of a temporary crown on tooth 2-2	60
8.	Removal of present restorations and decay on teeth 4-4 and 4-5	100
9.	Root canal treatments as needed	400–800
10.	Final filling on tooth 2-3 by your general dentist	
11.	Full-mouth scaling and polishing; review of oral hygiene methods	80
12.	Reassessment	80

Total estimated fee for [name of dentist] care   £1820–2220

Advanced Restorative Care (tentative plan)

1.	Possible additional periodontal surgery	0–975
2a.	Four to six tooth upper front bridge *or*	2000–3000
2b.	Two implant-supported crowns and a single crown on tooth 1-2	4300
3.	Cast metal posts and cores (as needed)	0–1200
4.	A three-toothed bridge on your upper right	1500
5.	A three-toothed bridge on your lower left	1500
6.	Crowns on teeth 4-4 and 4-5 if these can be saved	1000
7.	Replacement of crowns on your upper left and lower right	2000
8.	Fabrication of a night-time appliance	240

Total estimated fee for [name of dentist] care   £8240–12715

Maintenance Phase

1.	One hour hygienist maintenance every 3 months	(presently £60 per visit)
2	Annual comprehensive examinations	(presently £70 per year)

Summary

This estimate is for the services outlined and is based on surgical treatment completion within 2001, on payment of an implant deposit of £1200 three weeks before initial implant placement to cover costs of non-returnable components, and for other services at the time they are carried out.

Figure 5.4 A sample estimate of fees.

they are! Remember that patient costs are not solely the fees paid to the dentist. They may involve loss of income because of time off work, travel costs and perhaps childcare costs. Fees are presented for completeness of information on the options not for negotiation, although it is often feasible to modify the pace of treatment to spread costs. It is better to talk of a 'significant investment in treatment' rather than 'high costs' or 'expensive treatment'.

Many patients will spend more on an annual vacation (over in 2 weeks) or a second car (discarded in 3 or 4 years) than is proposed in even a complex treatment plan. Economists talk of 'opportunity cost' when considering the alternative ways in which a specific sum of money can be spent. Hence the discussion of proposed treatment should focus on why dental care offers more benefits and better long-term value than the alternative uses of the funds.

Where specific fees are not possible to determine, such as when the dentist is proposing complex crown and bridgework that may involve endodontics on some of the abutment teeth, it is better to quote a range of fees: from best possible to worst possible scenario to cover likely eventualities. We should bear in mind that 20–25% of teeth prepared for full-crown restorations subsequently require endodontics and, at the least, incorporate this likelihood into our estimates. Most of us would be unhappy if we were quoted a price of £14 000 for a new car and then find that the final total cost is £15 000. We would likely be happier if having been quoted up to £15 500 the final bill was £15 000. This psychology applies equally to our patients in the dental environment.

When quoting a fee, a time limit for the offer should be included, and the quote should clarify when payment is expected (Fig. 5.4). It should also clarify any aspects of treatment that are not included in the estimate, such as endodontics, periodontal surgery or implant surgery being referred to a specialist and it should encourage the patient to obtain estimates for these aspects of their proposed care.

Patients want to know how much treatment will cost, how long it is likely to take and when they are expected to pay. This is more than reasonable and dentists should provide this information routinely. The establishment of fees is discussed in detail in Chapter 7.

DELIVERING THE SERVICE OFFERED

Amsterdam (1979) said: 'If we are as happy with the fee when we have completed treatment as when we quote it, we have come out ahead'. Although dentists are seldom formally trained in marketing, many post-graduate courses focus on effective case presentation and achieving high levels of acceptance to treatment proposals. Fewer courses focus on the successful delivery of treatment once the plan has been accepted, and yet it is fundamental that the dentist should be able to 'deliver' the care that has been 'sold' to the patient.

Apart from the legal, moral and ethical obligations associated with offering to undertake a specific treatment plan for a patient, there is a sound business basis for ensuring that treatment is completed effectively. Successful general dentistry is reliant on a return trade with established patients, and with patient recommendations to potential new patients. Studies have shown that patients are seven times more likely to discuss a negative than a positive dental experience.

No dental fee, even for the most complex treatment plan, will generate sufficient income to retire and hide for the rest of one's life and so it is in everyone's interest that treatment has a successful outcome, not only at the point of completion but for an agreed follow-up period.

Most undergraduate dental programmes impart a sound education in the provision of a range of basic care. Continuing dental education and experience should allow the interested dentist to develop these skills in order progressively to manage more complex situations. It is not realistic, however, to move on to a full mouth reconstruction after completing three 3-unit bridges and a weekend course. It is dangerous to undertake surgical placement of implants, particularly in relation to vital structures, with a vague recollection of head and neck anatomy, 2 days in a hotel and the encouragement of a salesman. The discussion in Chapter 4, on when to work with a specialist, should be considered when complex treatment plans are developed. It is better for the patient, safer for the dentist and ultimately more rewarding for all if the dentist sees himself or herself as a key member in a dental team, rather than as a 'Jack, or Jill, of all trades'.

Ongoing self-appraisal is fundamental to the growth and development of any dentist, but the self-appraisal should not be based on a 'gut feeling' of treatment outcomes, but at least in part on a formal audit or peer review. It is human nature, described by psychologists as cognitive dissonance, for an individual to justify and rationalise past actions and choices on the basis that good people do not do bad things. At the same time, dentists have, in the past, had limited training on applying an evidence base, and too often new techniques have been accepted based more on the presentation skills of a speaker than the quality of the available research information. It is not unnatural then for a dentist to speak with enthusiasm about a course attended or a new piece of equipment purchased, but to be less forthcoming with colleagues when a technique is found to be disappointing or the equipment is gathering dust in a cupboard. Too often last year's technique or equipment-based courses are followed by this year's second-hand equipment advertisements in dental journals.

WARRANTIES AND GUARANTEES

With the growth in patient expectations and consumerism, patients are more likely to expect some form of formal guarantee for more advanced or expensive types of treatment. Among the factors that should be considered in offering any form of guarantee are:

- normal life expectancy of the type of treatment
- the patient's level of compliance with oral hygiene and attendance
- is the treatment accepted an 'ideal' or 'compromise' choice?
- the dentist's goodwill
- the likely form and costs of re-treatment; it is one thing to replace a fractured crown, another to manage a split root on a post crown with an extraction and implant-supported crown
- assistance in warranties by laboratories, implant companies or other manufacturers
- warranties and guarantees offered by competitors.

Ultimately, it is up to the dentist to decide what is fair and reasonable in any given situation. At the very least, the likely prognosis of various treatment options should be outlined in the treatment plan letter to the patient, and, if a problem arises, the dentist should weigh the goodwill created by standing by one's work against the illwill resulting from applying substantial additional charges to an already disappointed patient.

OFFERING TREATMENT CHOICES

This chapter has described the nuts and bolts of presenting treatment plan options to patients. It is extremely important to realise that not all patients will agree to the 'ideal' treatment proposed. Fear, limited available time, lack of funds or a more important immediate need for funds, such as childrens' education, may prevent the patient from agreeing to proceed with the advised treatment. It is easy to become disheartened when a carefully developed treatment plan is rejected. This may tempt dentists back to just listing fillings and calling this a treatment plan, or to planning only within the parameters set by third parties, who have never seen the patient. Dentists should remember that many who are at the top of their own profession have only a limited success rate. Pele failed to score on over 35% of the football games in which he played. Tiger Woods loses many more tournaments than he wins. Fran Tarkington, who holds the record for most successfully completed passes by a quarterback in American football, also holds the record for the most

unsuccessfully completed passes! But nobody thinks about the latter record.

By developing alternative treatment plans for a patient, the dentist gives the patient a choice and is

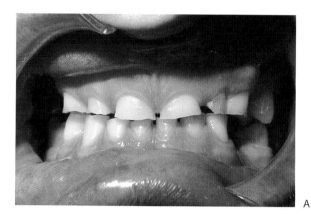

A

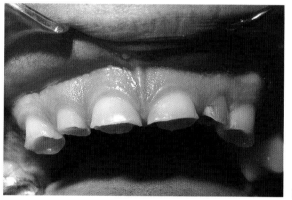

B

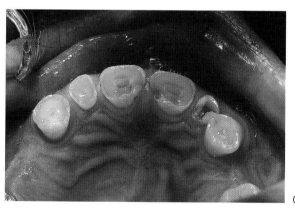

C

Figure 5.5 Patient K: offering treatment options. (A) The patient had advanced attrition and loss of vertical dimension, associated with a bruxing habit. He was concerned about the appearance of his teeth. (B,C) Close ups of the upper incisors show advanced tooth wear with compensatory deposition of secondary dentine. All teeth remain vital except for tooth 2-2, which has had a previous root canal treatment.

more likely to have one of the alternatives accepted. Provided the patient is happy with treatment, they may return later for 'ideal' treatment. This approach can be illustrated by the final treatment plan chosen by Patient K. This 49-year-old man presented for a second opinion with advanced attrition, and loss of vertical dimension, associated with a bruxing habit (Fig. 5.5). He was concerned about the appearance of his teeth. He had been advised in two previous consultations that a full mouth rehabilitation was the treatment of choice. The patient did not recall any alternative being presented, and he failed to return for the proposed treatment. When he presented to the author, again full mouth rehabilitation was advised, at a virtually identical fee to previous consultations, but two other options were also given. The patient decided on the partial overdenture option shown in Figures 5.6–5.9. The patient liked the improved appearance

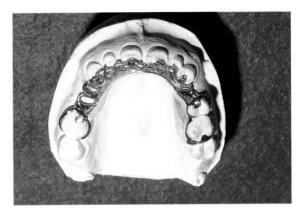

Figure 5.7 A chrome cobalt frame was made and fit for Patient K confirmed.

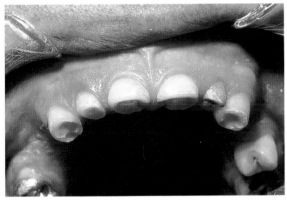

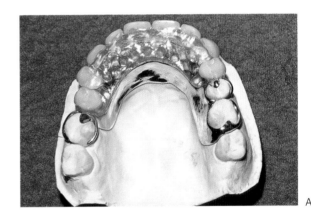

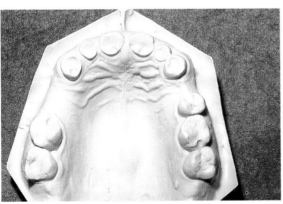

Figure 5.6 Patient K choses a partial denture. Preparation of the upper anterior teeth for a metal-based partial upper overdenture after 8 weeks of successful wear of an upper anterior bite plane. (B) Multiple prepared rest seats.

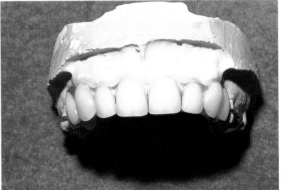

Figure 5.8 After an approved cosmetic try-in, the overdenture was processed in clear acrylic. This was chosen to allow the patient's own tissue colour to show through labially between the denture teeth.

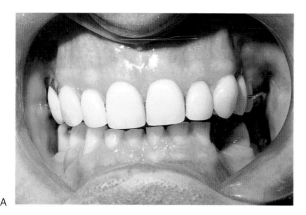

A

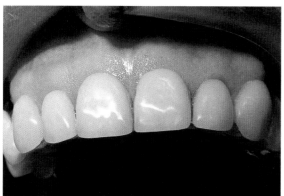

B

and was extremely happy with the compromise treatment plan carried out. He continued to wear the bite plane at night to protect the prepared teeth and avoid denture fracture. By offering alternative treatments, the dentist enabled the patient to feel comfortable with the practice and to agree to a reasonable compromise treatment. If in the future, the patient decides to move on to a fixed restorative option, it is unlikely that he will return to the practices that gave him no choices.

All dentists should be prepared to present patients with all reasonable options and not be disappointed, or take it personally, if proposals are not immediately taken up by every patient. Equally, if rejection rates outnumber acceptance of even compromise treatment plans, the dentist must examine presentation techniques and critically assess reasons for their failures. Here, the assistance of an experienced colleague or practice management consultant is often invaluable.

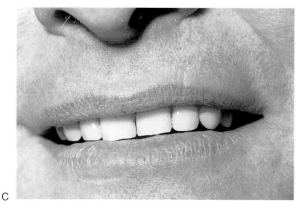

C

Figure 5.9 Patient K has the final overdenture inserted and is very happy with the improved appearance. Compromise treatment plan.

6 Sequence of treatment: a phased approach

When the house is on fire you don't send for a carpenter

While every patient is different, and specific clinical situations may well dictate modifications in treatment sequencing, there are some fundamental principles in planning the order in which treatment is provided. In general, treatment should follow the following sequence.

1. Relief of pain and other emergencies
2. Cause-related therapy
3. Reassessment
4. Basic corrective care
5. Reassessment
6. Prereconstructive therapy
7. Reconstructive therapy
8. Recall and maintenance care.

We will address each of these in turn, focusing not only on the individual stages but also on the inter-relationship between each.

RELIEF OF PAIN AND OTHER EMERGENCIES

Following the analogy of the opening quote; a fire needs a fire engine not a fire prevention officer. The relief of pain and approach to other emergencies includes:

- pulp extirpation
- caries removal and sedative dressing
- extraction
- irrigation and mouthwash
- prescription
- advice for reducing muscle and joint pain: soft diet, moist heat, and symmetrical exercises
- temporary soft splint for joint and muscle problems

- re-cementation of crowns, bridges and other restorations.

These may well precede definitive treatment planning but must not be performed in total isolation from planning the patient's care. Hence pulp extirpation of a tooth of doubtful prognosis is reasonable, but completion of endodontics only to find that the tooth cannot be restored or is periodontally hopeless is poor practice. Hopeless teeth should be extracted, preserving as much bone as possible to avoid creation of an aesthetic ridge defect and to keep open the option of implant placement.

We must remember that the patient's first impression of the quality of care in a practice will often be based on management of an emergency visit. Effective and prompt relief of pain is one of the most effective practice builders, whereas failure to relieve pain will cause the patient to rush to judgement on the overall skills of the dentist, and it is likely to lead them to seek future treatment elsewhere.

If someone is in pain, they do not want to be lectured on their own inadequacies, which have led to the problem. Hence it is inappropriate to point out that they should have come sooner, that their plaque control is poor or that their diet is at fault. Preventive advice should be restricted to what to expect and appropriate aftercare for the procedure carried out.

- *'The tooth will probably be a bit tender for a few days. Let me know if it doesn't settle by Monday.'* If it is tender for a few days, you have given accurate advice; if there is no pain you are obviously a skilled dentist; if the pain persists the patient knows what to do.

- *'Keep away from very hot and cold things for a few days: warm beer and cold coffee!'* If they forget and are exposed to extremes of temperature they may get a twinge, which will remind them of your skill in predicting the future. Attaching types of drink at unusual temperatures to this advise will stick in the patient's memory and help to reinforce the message.

- *'You should avoid hard or sticky foods where the temporary dressing has been placed.'* If they do pull out a dressing with chewing gum, you have again been shown to be able to predict their dental future; if not, you are still seen to be thorough and skilled.

- *'You should minimising smoking after the extraction since it can lead to a painful socket.'* Clearly a patient who is addicted to nicotine will have a hard time stopping, having just undergone the stress of toothache followed by an extraction; however, by offering the advice we both cover ourselves medico-legally and, if they do return with a dry socket smelling of cigarettes, we have again been seen as accurate in predicting a likely outcome. Either way, the clinician will create a favourable impression with the patient.

- *'Take the prescribed pain pills/antibiotics as it says on the bottle.'* Again, if they follow instructions all should be fine, while if they do not, the dentist has covered medico-legal aspects.

It is appropriate to leave them with parting encouragement:

> You've got a few ticking time bombs in there. Once you're over this, let's sit down and check over your mouth in detail, so that we can come up with a plan to avoid you having similar problems in the future.

This, combined with effective relief of pain is likely to bring the patient back for more comprehensive care. To cement the new relationship, a follow-up phone call to the patient either from the dentist or a member of staff will generally be greatly appreciated and may occasionally identify a problem that the patient did not like to call about. It can also be used to reinforce postoperative instructions. Most importantly, it has likely not been something the patient experienced in the past and can only create an impression of empathy and thoroughness.

Pulp extirpation

Pulp extirpation, provided it is carried out thoroughly, will generally assist in pain relief. Once confident that all pulpal tissue has been removed, the dentist must determine if drainage of pus is present. In the presence of a significant apical swelling, it is important to establish drainage. If copious drainage is achieved via the access preparation, incision of the swelling will likely not be needed; however, time must be allowed for drainage to occur. Hence a limited period of leaving the access preparation open to drain may well be indicated. This should not be the endpoint of emergency treatment. It is essential that the patient be advised on how to keep the access preparation open, generally by rinsing after meals. A follow-up appointment must also be made to reassess the swelling and drainage and to determine if the canal can be irrigated, medicated and sealed. Since there is a likelihood of the patient failing to keep this appointment if pain has been relieved, they should be advised of the short-term nature of opening the tooth, and a follow-up phone call must be made if they miss the appointment.

Caries removal and sedative dressing

Caries removal and sedative dressing carried out in the right circumstances can not only relieve pain quickly but also arrest caries progression and effectively buy time until treatment planning can be completed. Provided no pulp exposure is identified, then a reduction in the symptoms of reversible pulpitis is predictable, and the patient should gain rapid relief of pain. It is important that the dentist takes sufficient time and care to ensure that the dressing will be retained within the tooth until the next visit; hence where insufficient mechanical retention is available, the use of a stainless steel band or adhesive material is indicated. Too often the operator attempts a rushed type of restoration, which stands little chance of staying in place. Not only will this defeat the purpose of protecting the pulp, but it will create a poor first impression.

The patient in Figure 6.1a presented with multiple dental problems: toothache from 1-3 and 4-5 cervical, several other active carious lesions, periodontitis with spontaneous bleeding from the gingiva as well as several missing teeth, poor oral hygiene and diabetes. It is very difficult to place high-quality cervical composites until the periodontal condition has been controlled and plaque control will be ineffective while open carious lesions and pain remain. The first step, therefore, was to address her pain. Reinforced ZOE dressings were placed in all deep lesions after caries removal. Seven months later (Fig. 6.1b) the dressings were still in place but oral hygiene was much better and active periodontal treatment was complete. Conditions were then much better for placement of good-quality fillings.

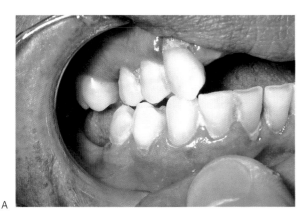

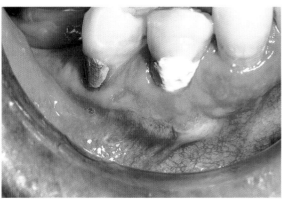

A

B

Figure 6.1 A patient with multiple dental problems. (A) The patient had toothache from 1-3 and 4-5 cervical, several other active carious lesions, periodontitis with spontaneous bleeding from the gingiva, several missing teeth, poor oral hygiene and diabetes. (B) Seven months later the dressings are still in place, but oral hygiene is much better and active periodontal treatment is complete. Conditions are ideal for placement of good-quality composite fillings.

Extraction

If it is clear that a painful tooth cannot be restored, or if extraction is considered to be a reasonable compromise approach, then it is best to proceed to this as soon as possible. Once it has been confirmed that the patient's medical history is clear, the operator should review a current radiograph of the tooth and, provided there is sufficient time available and the dentist is comfortable that the extraction is within their capabilities, effective local anaesthesia should be obtained and the tooth extracted. Significant future planning is involved in both the decision to extract and the extraction itself. The patient should have been informed of the sequelae of tooth loss in addition to the normal postoperative instructions and possible

complications; these include possible overeruption of opposing teeth and tipping of adjacent teeth, which may eventually compromise future tooth replacements. Where appropriate, changes in function, aesthetics and phonetics should also be discussed.

A phone call that evening to ensure that the patient is both comfortable and following instructions will go a long way to establishing a good dentist/patient relationship—and will often be discussed favourably with the patient's friends.

Irrigation and mouthwash

When a patient presents with an acute soft tissue problem such as pericoronitis, acute gingivitis or a traumatic ulcer, the dentist will often limit treatment to irrigation of the site and/or advising a mouthwash such as chlorhexidine. It is important to advise the patient on the likelihood of relief, the time frame within which it is expected and what to do if things do not improve. Possible necessary future treatment if pain persists, as well as follow-up treatment once relief has been obtained, should be discussed. Again a follow-up phone call, likely by a staff member, will create a positive impression with the patient and may identify the stoic who does not wish to bother the dentist, even though things are not improving.

Prescription

A prescription should only be issued after careful examination and diagnosis of a patient's problem, not as a substitute for these: overuse of antibiotics is pandemic, analgesic abuse is too common, drug intolerance and resistance is increasing and there can be no excuse for inappropriate prescription of drugs. When a prescription is indicated, the patient's current medical history must be reviewed for possible allergies, interactions or other contraindications and the patient must be advised of the appropriate regimen to follow. Again the dentist should give some indication of the likelihood of relief, the time frame within which it is expected and what to do if things do not improve. A careful record of what has been prescribed should be kept and compliance confirmed on the next visit.

Advice on reducing muscle and joint pain

Myofacial and joint pain can often be alleviated with a soft diet, moist heat, and symmetrical exercises for joint and muscle problems.

When a patient presents on emergency with myofacial or temporomandibular joint pain, then the dentist's first priority is the accurate diagnosis of the condition and the second is the rapid relief of discomfort where this is possible. Appropriate examination of joints and muscles of mastication has been outlined in Chapter 2. Where joint function is normal with a full range of opening and lateral movements free of disc displacement, and discomfort is limited to some of the muscles of mastication, it is often sufficient to place the patient on a soft diet, institute moist heat application (damp facecloths either heated with warm water or microwaved till warm) over the affected muscles and initiate gentle symmetrical opening and closing exercises. The patient should be encouraged to apply this moist heat prior to times of heavy use of the mouth: in other words, before eating, before sleeping when nocturnal bruxism is likely, before any prolonged talking (as with a lecturer or teacher) and, of course, before any long dental appointment. It is indeed unwise to attempt anything beyond simple urgent dental treatment when a patient has acute myofascial pain. Even where treatment is essential, moist heat breaks during long appointments can head off unneeded exacerbations of the problem. It can be explained to the patient that the heat application and exercises before using the jaw are like the warm-up exercises of an athlete before any major exertion, or anyone doing a warm-up before aerobics or running.

Where disc displacement has occurred and the patient is diagnosed as having anterior disc displace-ment with reduction, the opening exercises may initially have to take place in a more protrusive position, where the disc is recaptured and click-free opening can occur. It is generally found that, provided the patient is faithful in carrying out the heat and exercise regimen, not only is discomfort reduced but the timing of the click becomes earlier or may disappear completely. More details of appropriate management of these problems can be found in Okeson (1985).

Temporary splints for joint and muscle problems

Where wear facets and hypertonic muscles are present in conjunction with myofascial and/or joint pain, some form of occlusal splint may be indicated. It is generally accepted that a full-arch Michigan type splint, made of hard processed acrylic, offers the best opportunity of pain relief with the least risk of complications. In most practice situations, it will take several days to have a laboratory processed splint made. As a short-term means of pain relief, some practitioners find a soft occlusal splint, essentially a sports mouthguard, can give the patient some initial improvement.

Where a practice has an in-house vacuum former and can make such an appliance within the day of patient presentation, this may be a reasonable temporary measure until a hard acrylic appliance is made. It may also be a short-term treatment where the dentist has identified a specific acute situation, likely to be self-limiting, where longer-term appliance use is not likely. This may be a patient experiencing facial pain because of clenching around final examinations, the death of a loved one or similar situations. The soft splint must not be considered to be a long-term appliance. It is by its nature of even thickness, thus creating initial contacts posteriorly and seldom giving anterior contact. The nature of the material makes it impossible to adjust to establish balanced contact. More alarmingly, if worn for an extended period of time, the appliances almost invariably perforates posteriorly, resulting in uncontrolled occlusal contacts and even irreversible tooth movement.

The advent of strong light-cured materials such as Triad enables the dentist or a well-trained auxiliary to fabricate a hard Michigan type splint in around an hour within the practice. As this technology becomes more widely available, the indications for a temporary soft splint are likely to be restricted to sports mouth-guards. Figure 6.2 shows the manufacture of such a splint by a dental auxiliary. It was inserted and adjusted for the patient within 2 hours of initial impression taking.

Re-cementation of crowns, bridges and other restorations

It has been said that there are two kinds of dentist in this world: the kind that, when a crown comes out, sticks it back in and the kind who work out why it came out in the first place.

Often the dentist's first contact with a new patient is when they present on an emergency basis with a crown or onlay out or a bridge loose or out. While this may well happen when the dentist is busy, has other patients waiting and has limited time available, for the

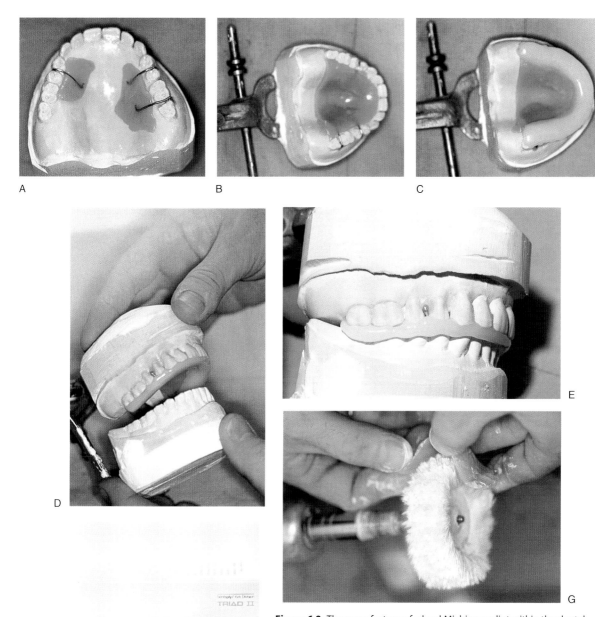

Figure 6.2 The manufacture of a hard Michigan splint within the dental practice. (A) The upper model is coated with separating agent and pre-made ball clasps are bent to fit and embedded in Triad denture material. (B) The rest of the palate is covered and this part of the splint can now be partly light cured. (C) After applying bonding agent, clear Triad is added to the occlusal surfaces of the teeth to a thickness of 2 to 4 mm. (D) The hinge articulator has been set to a retruded arc of closure wax bite taken at an increased vertical dimension of approximately 4 mm in the incisor region. The articulator is closed until the lower teeth make imprints in the uncured Triad. (It is also possible to carry out this stage in the patient's mouth and avoid the need for articulating the models.) (E) With the articulator in the closed position, excess material is trimmed and any additions made to correct deficiencies. (F) The appliance is light cured for 4 to 6 minutes. (G) The appliance is polished before trying in the patient's mouth. A final polish occurs after adjustment to establish the desired occlusal scheme.

patient it is their only dental contact that day, that week or perhaps even that year. If the crown has been out several times in the past, the dentist has two choices: to repeat the treatment and likely errors of the past dentists (and be categorised with former dentists in the patient's eyes) or to work out why the crown is coming out repeatedly, inform the patient of reason(s) for the problem, correct them immediately where possible and arrange to correct them later where immediate correction is not practical.

Among the factors that may cause displacement of a crown or bridge are:

- caries
- preparation too short
- preparation too tapered
- post too short
- vertical root fracture
- restoration does not fit or cement wash-out
- the occlusion is traumatic, usually in excursions but occasionally even in the intercuspal position
- lack of a mutually protected occlusion, usually anterior crowns with lack of posterior teeth
- lack of a mutually protected occlusion at night; a partial denture may provide mutual protection during the day but is removed at night, with no provision made for protection of anterior teeth.

Often, more than one of these factors exists at the same time. In order to make an informed diagnostic decision and give treatment recommendations, the clinician will usually need a periapical radiograph of the tooth and should put the restoration back in place and have the patient tap in the intercuspal position, then go through lateral and protrusive movements. If fremitus is felt in the restoration during any of these movements, it is likely that the restoration is exposed to forces that will displace it again. The radiograph will provide essential information to the clinician. Important factors to consider are:

- how long is the root?
- is there any periapical pathology?
- is there periradicular radiolucency, which is often indicative of root fracture?
- if a root canal filling is present, is it satisfactory?
- if the restoration is a post crown, does the post take full advantage of the available root length?

- is the post preparation within the root canal system or does it approach or perforate the outside of the root?

Based on clinical and radiographic assessment, the clinician must ask five questions.

1. *Is the restoration and tooth satisfactory in its present state?* If so, excess cement can be removed and the crown and tooth can be cleaned and the restoration re-cemented.

2. *Is the restoration satisfactory with minor modifications?* Where limited occlusal adjustment or the fabrication of a night splint is deemed as all that is needed, and the patient agrees to this, the dentist can proceed to re-cement after appropriate other treatment is initiated.

3. *Is the restoration beyond salvaging?* The post may be too short or the margins may be open either because of poor fit or caries. Provided the tooth itself has a good prognosis and the patient agrees, caries if present should be removed, a well-fitting provisional restoration should be made and appointments arranged for re-treatment, in the context of an overall treatment plan.

4. *Does the tooth itself need additional treatment before restoration retreatment is started?* It may well be that the tooth needs endodontics treatment or re-treatment, or that a periodontal flap for crown lengthening is required, before a new restoration can be made. In these situations, a provisional restoration or modification of the original restoration (on occasion relined with acrylic) can be made and cemented with temporary cement.

5. *Is the tooth unrestorable?* The presence of a root fracture, perforation or deep caries may render the tooth unrestorable. In this case the patient must be informed of the situation and of immediate and longer-term tooth replacement options. It may be permissible to re-cement the restoration temporarily until extraction and tooth replacement can be arranged, but this must only be considered a very short-term measure.

Whichever of the above situations prevail, it is of paramount importance that the patient is fully informed of the situation, of the prognosis and, where appropriate, of the temporary nature of the emergency treatment that has been carried out. Re-cementing a restoration with poor prognosis, more in hope than expectation of success, often in order to get the patient in and out quickly, is not only poor practice but, in the patient's eyes, appears to confirm that the dentist is 'assuming ownership and responsibility' of someone else's possibly inferior work. *Whoever touches it last takes the blame.* The dentist can clarify the situation not only by a clear explanation of the situation, but by reinforcing phrases such as, '*When* the crown comes out again, we should…' not '*If* the crown comes out again we might have to…'

The post crowns in Figure 6.3 had a history of coming out repeatedly. The post of the left (tooth 1-1) was short but a good root canal filling was present and it should be feasible to make a longer post and retreat the tooth with a good prognosis. The post on the right (tooth 2-1), although longer, extended into an area of internal root resorption and secondary root fracture. The prognosis for this tooth was hopeless and its extraction and subsequent replacement should be planned. Clearly the type of replacement for tooth 2-1 should be decided before the new restoration for 1-1 is completed.

In Figure 6.4 the post crown on the left (tooth 1-1) had been re-cemented on six occasions and subsequent review indicated that no radiographs had been taken since crowns were made 4 years previously. Because of increasing pain and swelling, the patient presented to a new dentist, whose radiographs showed not only a short post but also that both central incisors had been perforated, likely during post preparation. Both teeth were subsequently extracted.

CAUSE-RELATED THERAPY

The second phase of treatment should focus on the cause rather than the effects of disease. This phase includes:

- plaque control instruction
- diet counselling
- fluoride advice
- smoking cessation advice
- fissure sealing
- calculus removal and root planing
- dressing of active carious lesions
- removal of overhangs
- wearing appliances, as advised.

All aspects of cause-related therapy are designed to bring the patient to a level of understanding of the

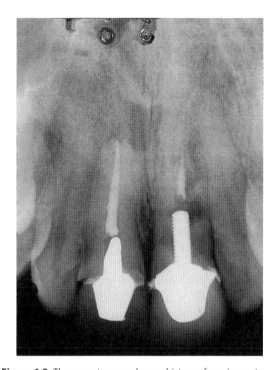

Figure 6.3 These post crowns have a history of coming out, and being re-cemented repeatedly. The post of the left (tooth 1-1) is short with a good root canal filling; it should be feasible to make a longer post and re-treat the tooth. The post on the right (tooth 2-1), although longer, extends into an area of internal root resorption and secondary root fracture. Its prognosis is hopeless.

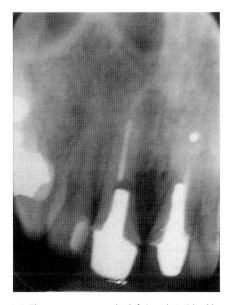

Figure 6.4 The post crown on the left (tooth 1-1) had been re-cemented on six occasions. A radiograph showed a short post and perforation of both central incisors.

disease processes and to being actively involved in their control and prevention.

While many of these preventive-based activities can effectively be delegated to the hygienist or other auxiliary, the dentist must not give the impression that these are being delegated because they are not important. An appropriate build up such as: 'I want you to see Catherine our hygienist to discuss home-care and the possibility of stopping smoking, because she has had special advanced training in these areas and can customise her advice to your individual situation' is likely to put the patient into the right frame of mind for the appointment.

If this visit follows a pain relief appointment, it is a huge positive step for the dentist to 'drop in' to see how things are going. It is even better if the dentist knows in advance how things are, because the front desk has already asked and relayed the information to the dentist. Then there are no surprises when he/she drops in.

INITIAL REASSESSMENT

It is important before embarking on even basic corrective care, to assess how things are going with regard to:

- prognosis of doubtful teeth
- initial compliance with homecare advice, and to
- finalise the basic treatment plan.

This may well be the visit at which comprehensive treatment planning and treatment options are developed. It will certainly allow the dentist to gauge the impact of initial cause-related advice and it is an appropriate time to establish the prognosis of doubtful teeth. The treatment options can then be discussed in an environment free of pain and in a preventive context. If the patient's preceding impressions of the dental team's empathy and skill have been favourable they are likely to feel 'I am in the right place' and be receptive to treatment proposals.

At this visit, the dentist must have readily to hand all necessary diagnostic data such as charting, study casts, radiographs. Having reassessed progress in preventive measures, it is appropriate to map out the next phase of treatment and discuss ultimate goals. It may well only be at this point that the dentist gets a feel for the patient's level of interest, and where the patient feels sufficiently comfortable to discuss specific dental concerns.

BASIC CORRECTIVE CARE

Basic corrective care will include:

- endodontics on teeth that are strategically important
- placement of plastic restorations
- placement of provisional crowns, bridges and interim dentures, especially where there is a need to address an aesthetic concern early in the treatment plan
- limited occlusal adjustment
- splinting of excessively mobile teeth
- use of occlusal appliances
- extraction of hopeless and non-strategic teeth
- periodontal surgery for pocket reduction or regenerative purposes.

All aspects of basic corrective care are designed to repair or minimise the damage caused by disease processes. This has been for many years the basic bread and butter area of general dental practice; however, when it is offered without an effective cause-related preventive plan, it has been the most disillusioning part of general practice, with patients returning year after year with recurrence of similar problems. It is important in more complex cases that this phase is completed thoroughly before the dentist and patient embark on more sophisticated types of treatment. Too often crowns, bridges and partial dentures are placed in a situation where the basic disease processes have not been arrested. It is also common for advanced restorative dentistry to be offered as a 'cure' for progressive disease. Figure 6.5 shows a 56-year-old patient whose chief complaint was the development of spacing between her upper anterior teeth. This was treated by the placement of three overwide crowns. Spacing continued to develop because the underlying causes (advancing periodontitis, deep bite and a lack of a stable posterior occlusion) were never mentioned, far less addressed. Her previous dentist had even suggested redoing the crowns at an even wider size. The treatment of *effect* without the management of *cause* is short term at best and inevitably leads to a recurrence of the original problem, as well as a resentful patient.

REASSESSMENT AFTER BASIC CORRECTIVE CARE

The reassessment after basic corrective care is especially important. It is used to:

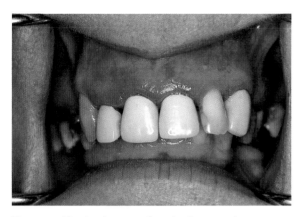

Figure 6.5 The development of spacing between the upper anterior teeth had been treated by the placement of three overwide crowns. Spacing continued to develop because the underlying causes were never addressed.

- assess ongoing compliance with homecare advice
- assess healing of any surgical procedures
- finalise the reconstructive treatment plan.

As with a diet, most patients do well with oral hygiene efforts and smoking cessation for the first few days, but many drop by the wayside after a few weeks and this point in the treatment plan may be used to attempt to remotivate those who have lapsed. If compliance is good, the treatment is at a point where the details of the reconstructive treatment plan can be finalised; if not, then it is appropriate to put the patient into a holding pattern, which may involve one or two hygiene recalls over a period of a few months to try to get them back on track. The need for this holding pattern will vary with the level of lapsed compliance as well as the complexity, risk and cost of advanced restorative plan. The dentist should have, by this point, achieved a stable functional and aesthetic dentition, all be it with basic materials, and there should be no rush to advanced care if compliance is doubtful. Over the years, dentists seldom regret going too slowly, but I have come across many situations where disappointment, failure and even litigation have resulted from going too quickly. Often the rush to definitive restorative care is merely a cover-up for inadequately made provisional restorations, or lack of attention to occlusal considerations. The dentist hopes, often in vain, that the 'permanent' restoration will be back before the provisional restoration breaks or falls out. In rushing ahead, the dentist loses the

potentially major advantage of learning from the provisional restoration: judging tissue response to crown contour, assessing if the preparation is retentive enough, determining if the pulp is reacting adversely to treatment to date and gaining patient feedback on contour of teeth.

It is perhaps the greatest weakness of many dental curricula that, if this reassessment even occurs, there is almost invariably a rush to carry out advanced procedures because of an over-riding time restriction or list of requirements. We do no service to students, patients or the profession by placing advanced restorations in doubtful situations. Academics must accept a considerable responsibility for poor practice in the general dental environment because of the examples set in dental school. Any student should be given more credit for saying 'No, this mouth is not ready' than for being coerced into placing crowns and bridges into dirty mouths.

PRERECONSTRUCTIVE THERAPY

At the prereconstruction stage, a number of basic therapies may be required to lay the groundwork for the final reconstruction:

- elective endodontics
- periodontal surgery for restorative purposes
  — crown lengthening
  — exposure of sound tooth structure
  — cosmetic periodontal procedures (see Chapter 10)
  — control of recession
  — vestibular deepening
- adjunctive orthodontic procedures
  — abutment alignment
  — forced eruption
  — rapid extrusion
- placement of endosseous dental implants.

Periodontal surgery for restorative purposes can have a number of objectives. Patient L was a young woman who had temporary bridges replacing congenitally missing lateral incisors. These had come off several times and she had been referred for crown lengthening prior to final impressions (Fig. 6.6). This was achieved by surgery to extend the 'biological width'; an area of root of around 3 mm beyond the crown margins above the bone crest (Fig. 6.7) as

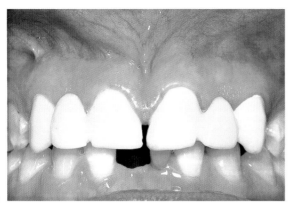

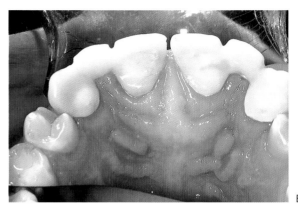

A   B

Figure 6.6 Patient L: prereconstruction surgery to lengthen crowns.

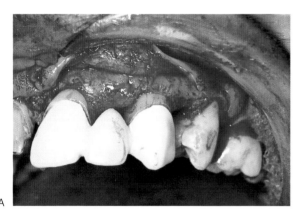

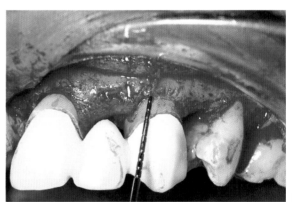

A   B

Figure 6.7 Retraction of a flap to show the area of root approximately 3 mm beyond the crown margins above the bone crest.

described by Ingber et al. (1977). The margins cannot be extended into this zone unless ostectomy is carried out to allow reformation of biological width at a more apical point (Fig. 6.8). The gingival margins should be allowed to heal for approximately 16-20 weeks before they are retracted for taking an impression (Fig. 6.9). Three months after the final bridges were placed, a favourable aesthetic result and gingival response had been achieved (Fig. 6.10). The missing lower teeth were replaced later—and the patient went on to become a dentist.

Figure 6.11 shows a patient for whom a 4-unit bridge was planned. However, an existing filling on the premolar extended considerably subgingival; when reduction for occlusal porcelain has been completed there would be little retentive crown length. For this patient, crown lengthening was achieved (Fig. 6.11C, D). The patient shown in Figure 6.12 has a treatment

plan that calls for new crowns on the lower canine and first premolar (teeth 4-3 and 4-4). Because of the combined effects of recession and a high muscle attachment, the gingival margin was unlikely to withstand the traumas of retraction and impression without worsening the mucogingival situation. There was also no room to allow use of an I-bar type clasp. The placement of a free gingival graft (Fig. 6.12B) stabilised the mucogingival situation and increased vestibular depth (Fig. 6.12C). After 4 months, it would be safe to proceed with the crowns and partial denture with predictable outcomes.

Figure 6.13 also illustrates periodontal surgery to control recession. A 3-unit bridge was planned to replace a missing lower second premolar (Fig. 6.13A). Recession was already present on both abutments and a high muscle attachment extends well onto the edentulous ridge (likely caused by a traumatic

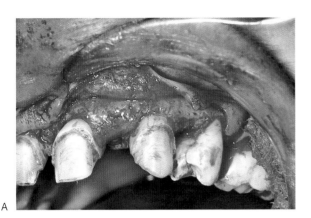

A

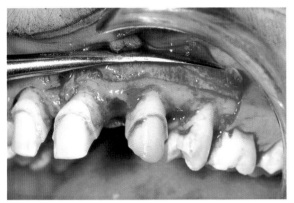

B

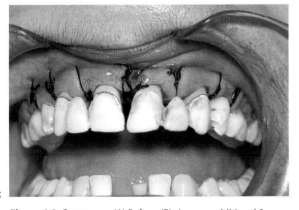

C

Figure 6.8 Ostectomy. (A) Before; (B) since an additional 3 mm of retentive crown length was desired, the corresponding amount of bone must be removed. (C) Flaps were apically positioned around 3 mm coronal to the new position of the osseous crest and sutured at that position using vertical mattress periosteal sutures. This allowed space for the maturation of a new biological width at this more apical position.

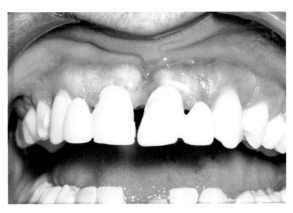

Figure 6.9 At 18 weeks the gingival margins are mature enough for an impression to be taken without adverse effect.

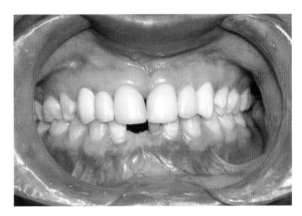

Figure 6.10 Patient L 3 months after bridge placement.

extraction). Not only is a stable gingival margin on the abutments unlikely, but oral hygiene measures under the pontic would also be difficult because of the muscle position. A free gingival graft, customised to fit the area, was taken from a palatal donor site and sutured in position after appropriate preparation of the recipient site. Care must be taken to identify and avoid the mental foramen and the exiting mental nerve (Fig. 6.13C). Healing at 6 weeks showed the establishment of a stable mucogingival complex (Fig. 6.13D). It was then feasible to fabricate a bridge with stable gingival margins and a pontic design that facilitated effective oral hygiene.

Periodontal surgery is also needed to achieve vestibular depth if this is inadequate. Because of the loss of all lower right teeth distal to the lateral incisor, partial denture design and retention was very difficult for the patient shown in Figure 6.14A. Implants were not an option for financial and anatomical reasons, and so a swinglock partial denture was the treatment of choice. As described in the literature, this technique requires 8 to 10 mm of buccal vestibular depth, and

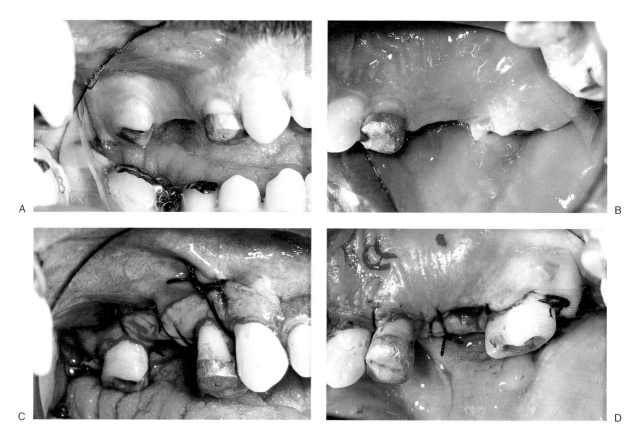

Figure 6.11 Exposure of sound tooth structure. (A,B) This patient has an existing filling on a premolar that extends subgingival and has little retentive crown length. (C,D) After completion of an apically positioned flap with necessary ostectomy, sound tooth structure was exposed and ample retentive crown length was made available.

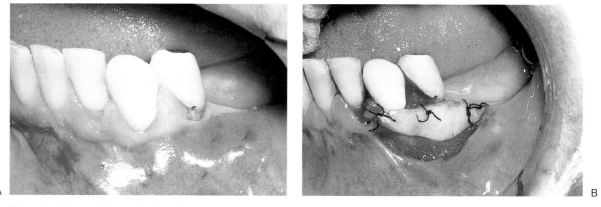

Figure 6.12 Control of recession. (A) The gingival margin in this patient was unlikely to withstand the traumas of retraction and impressions. (B) Placement of a free gingival graft to stabilise the mucogingival situation and increase vestibular depth.   *Continued*

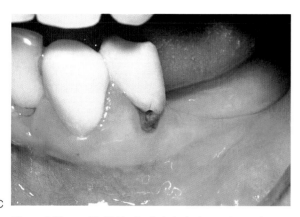

C

Figure 6.12, cont'd (C) The healed gingival complex ready to proceed to crowns.

the patient had little more than 3 mm available. The vestibule can be deepened surgically and a recipient bed prepared for an extensive free gingival graft (Fig. 6.14B). Since the patient wore a complete upper denture, all donor tissue can be obtained from under the denture and a soft lining added during healing. The graft here was carefully sutured in place using a continuous sling horizontal mattress periosteal suture to maximise the binding down of the graft (Fig. 6.14C). Once the graft has matured (Fig. 6.15A, B) the swing-lock partial denture can be fabricated (Fig. 6.16A). There was now adequate space for the full closure of the labial component without impingement onto labial muscle attachments (Fig. 6.16B).

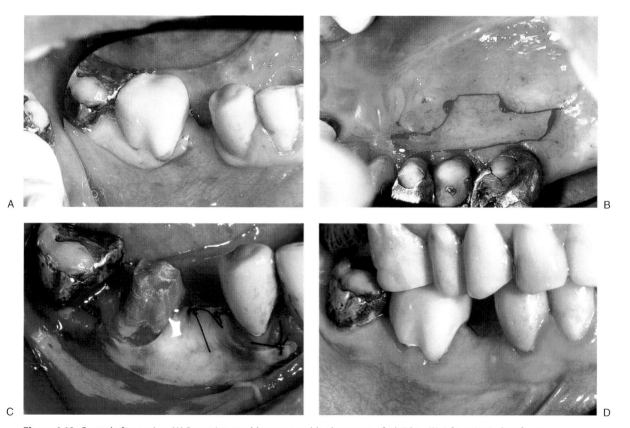

A

B

C

D

Figure 6.13 Control of recession. (A) Recession would prevent stable abutments of a bridge. (B) A free gingival graft was customised to fit the area from a palatal donor site. (C) The graft was sutured into position. (D) The healed mucogingival complex.

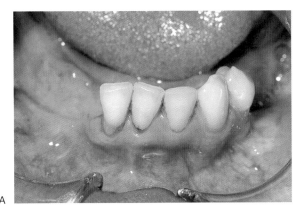

A

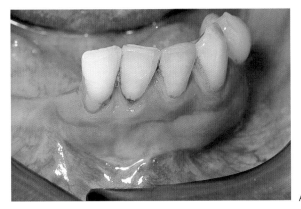

A

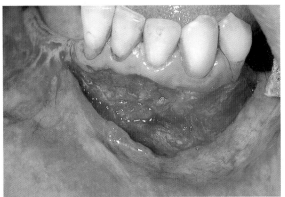

B

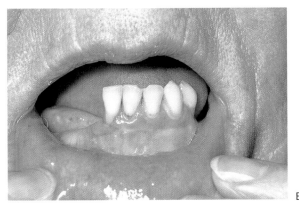

B

Figure 6.15 The matured graft now has adequate vestibular depth.

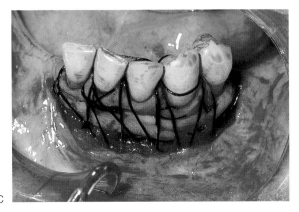

C

Figure 6.14 Vestibular deepening. (A) The patient had approximately 3 mm buccal vestibular depth and needed 8–10 mm for a swinglock partial denture. (B) The vestibule was deepened surgically. (C) A graft was sutured in place using a continuous sling horizontal mattress periosteal suture.

This phase also includes cosmetic periodontal procedures (Ch. 10) and adjunctive orthodontic procedures such as molar uprighting, abutment alignment, forced eruption and rapid extrusion. All of these orthodontic procedures can improve both the aesthetics and long-term prognosis of advanced restorative care.

Figure 6.17 illustrates the orthodontic uprighting of a molar prior to fixed bridgework. While it may technically be possible to parallel this tooth with an anterior abutment or use some type of attachment to make bridge placement possible, there is a great risk of pulp exposure on the mesial, and the distal preparation will inevitably be short with limited retention and risk of cement wash-out. As the tooth becomes upright, the preparation can be less tapered; the pulp is less threatened and loading is down the long axis of the tooth. Figures 6.18 and 6.19 illustrate mesial uprighting of a tipped premolar. The patient presented with a distally tipped premolar, overeruption of several teeth and a desire to eliminate her partial denture for functional and aesthetic reasons. With a combination of localised fixed and removable orthodontics and ongoing occlusal adjustment, the premolar was gradually uprighted mesially, paralleling

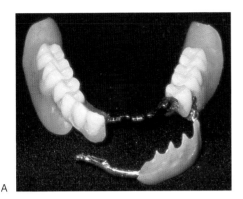

A

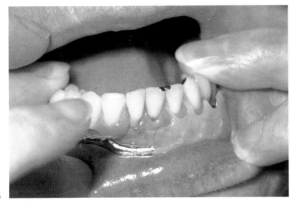

B

Figure 6.16 Swinglock partial denture. (A) Fabrication of the denture. (B) The increase in vestibular depth achieved with the graft (Figs 6.14 and 6.15) allowed full closure of the denture without impinging on the labial muscle attachments. (Prosthesis by Dr R. Brygider, Nova Scotia, Canada.)

it to the other potential abutments and opening the pontic space (Fig. 6.18B, C). Once the premolar was in position, the teeth could be prepared and the final bridge made with appropriate pontic size and embrasure spaces (Fig. 6.19).

Mesial drift often compromises embrasures between teeth and complicates impression taking and subsequent patient homecare. Figures 6.20–6.23 illustrate a case where orthodontic root separation was used to open the embrasure between the molar teeth. This not only allowed the taking of accurate impressions but also the creation of ideal embrasures to facilitate homecare. The patient presented with a failing bridge, significant periodontal bone loss on the mesial of the first molar and a major root proximity problem between the molars, which made impression taking and oral hygiene difficult. After scaling, root planning and mesial bone grafting, the teeth were prepared to receive provisional restorations (Fig. 6.21).

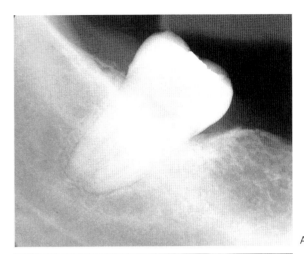

A

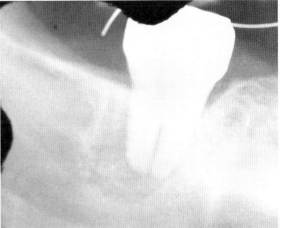

B

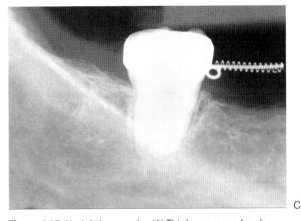

C

Figure 6.17 Uprighting a molar. (A) This lower second molar has tipped mesially because of the loss of the first molar. It presents at 45 degrees to the anterior abutment and with a mesial infrabony defect. (B) As the tooth uprights and erupts, mesial bone remodels and more tooth structure is available for crown retention. (C) With the tooth in position, mesial bone has fully remodelled, the abutments are parallel and a classical 3-unit bridge preparation is possible.

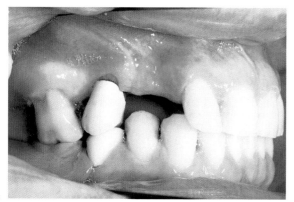

A

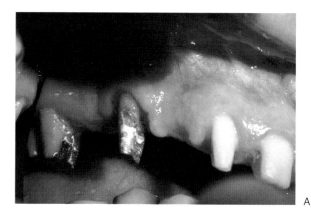

A

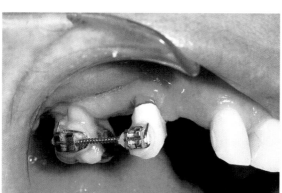

B

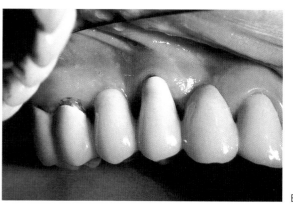

B

Figure 6.19 Preparation of teeth for the final bridge after successful mesial uprighting (Fig. 6.18).

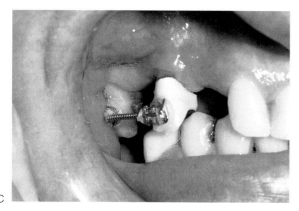

C

Figure 6.18 Mesial uprighting. (A) There is a distally tipped premolar and overeruption of several teeth. (B, C) Localised fixed and removable orthodontics to adjust the premolar, paralleling it to other potential bridge abutments and opening pontic space.

The provisional restorations were made and two brackets, a straight wire and an open coil spring were placed. The second molar was taken out of occlusion to facilitate its movement. Within 6 weeks, the second molar had moved sufficiently distally to allow refinement of tooth preparation and final impression

taking (Fig. 6.22). The final bridge was then made with ideal embrasure spaces, facilitating optimum oral hygiene and maintenance (Fig. 6.23) and enhanced long-term prognosis.

When a tooth fracture extends far subgingivally (Fig. 6.24) access for preparation and impression taking is often impossible. Although periodontal crown lengthening is always an option, this can cause significant aesthetic problems for a single anterior tooth and can compromise bone support for adjacent teeth. The use of orthodontic **rapid extrusion** is possible to bring down a fractured tooth to a position where restoration is possible without compromising anterior aesthetics. This technique is a variation of forced eruption first described by Ingber (1974, 1976, 1989) to modify the topography of periodontal infrabony defects (see Figs 6.24–6.26 and 10.17). Heavy forces are used to extrude the tooth rapidly from its alveolus. Even with such forces, it may be necessary to sever the periodontal ligament under local anaesthetic

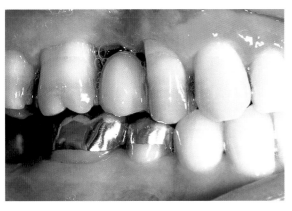

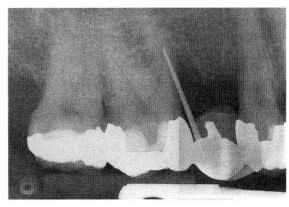

A   B

Figure 6.20 Patient M: orthodontic root separation. (A) Presentation with failing bridge, periodontal bone loss on the mesial of the first molar and a root proximity problem between the molars. (B) Radiograph with silver point to illustrate the depth of the infrabony defect.

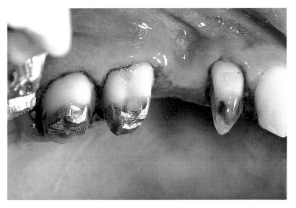

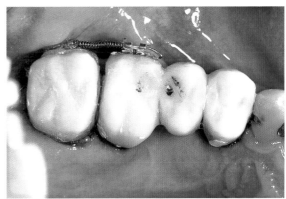

A   B

Figure 6.21 Patient M. (A) Preparation of the teeth to receive provisional restorations. Note the very limited space between the molars. (B) Provisional restorations with two brackets, a straight wire and an open spring.

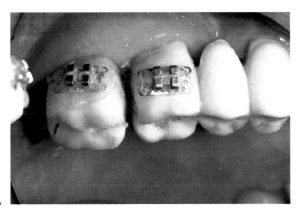

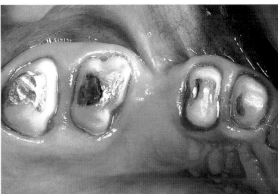

A   B

Figure 6.22 Patient M after 6 weeks. The second molar has moved distally sufficient to allow tooth preparation.

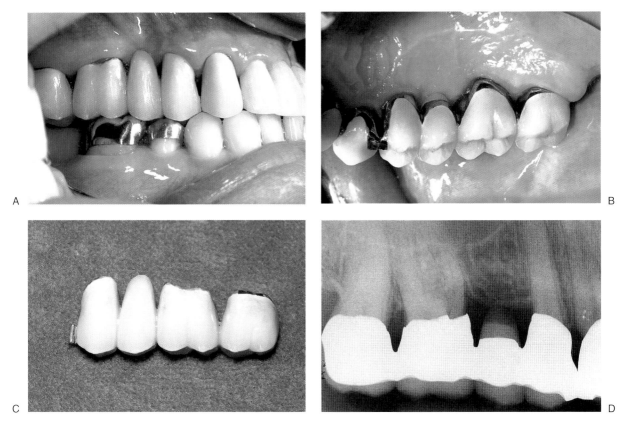

A

B

C

D

Figure 6.23 Patient M's final bridge. (A–C) There are ideal embrasure spaces. (D) The final radiograph shows the development of bone between the molars where the teeth have been separated, as well as a successful bone graft on the mesial of the molar. (Periodontal treatment described in Figs 6.20–6.23 was by Dr Tony Rose, Washington DC.)

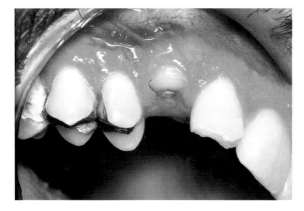

Figure 6.24 Patient N: orthodontic rapid extrusion for an upper canine that has fractured 5 mm subgingivally on the palatal side.

to prevent the tissue and bone erupting with the tooth. Once tooth movement has been completed and access has been gained to the palatal, final tooth preparation can be carried out and impressions taken (Fig. 6.26).

Since the early 1990s, the prereconstructive phase has expanded to include the placement of endosseous dental implants. Figures 6.27 and 6.28 show the placement of four titanium implants in the incisor area in conjunction with extraction of two lateral incisors fractured by trauma. Patient O already had a 4-unit bridge replacing both central incisors, which was also damaged in the fall. In order to avoid a partial denture, the patient opted for an immediate temporary resin-retained bridge (Fig. 6.29). Other aspects of the patient's pre-reconstructive treatment can be completed during the period that the implants remain buried. The final reconstruction involved implant integration and exposure and completion of the crowns. These are splinted so that the restoration will survive even if one or even two implants fail at some future time (Fig. 6.30).

This is also a time when decisions should be made on the need for elective endodontics, particularly on teeth with large restorations, limited tooth structure

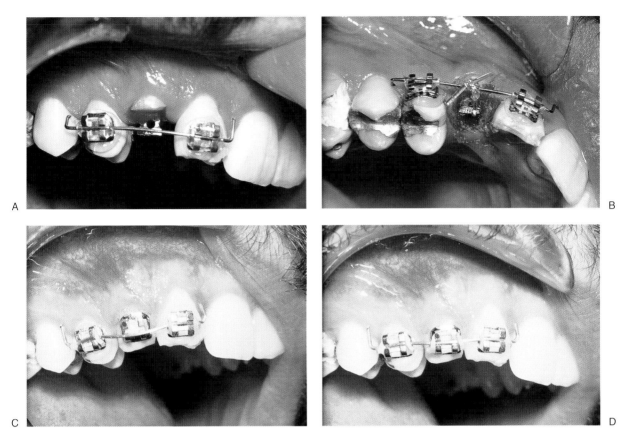

Figure 6.25 Patient N: orthodontic rapid extrusion. (A, B) A modified Parapost was locked into the canal using Durelay and initially linked to an archwire by use on an elastic ligature. The Durelay ensures good post retention while allowing for its eventual removal as part of tooth preparation. (C, D) After initial movement, composite is added to the post and a bracket placed. Heavy forces are used to rapidly extrude the tooth from its alveolus.

and a past history of pain. Where these teeth are to become crown or bridge abutments, then serious consideration should be given to the relative ease of performing endodontics at this point compared with the possible complexity of performing it later.

With all of these prereconstructive treatments, appropriate healing times must be allowed before embarking on the reconstructive phase. This would generally mean at least 4 weeks after endodontics, up to 20 weeks after periodontal surgery in the cosmetic zone and, depending on the implant protocol followed, between 3 and 6 months before implants receive the definitive restoration. With adjunctive orthodontics, some interim plan for retention is essential until the advanced restorative phase is carried out.

RECONSTRUCTIVE THERAPY

Reconstructive therapy includes:

- crowns
- bridges
- metal-based partial dentures
- implant-supported restorations.

This stage will involve the fabrication and placement of all definitive restorations (generally those involving laboratory assistance). If it is approached in a phased treatment sequence such as described here, then few surprises should be expected. The use of well-made temporary partial dentures and provisional fixed restorations should have provided a 'dress rehearsal' to eliminate potential problems effectively

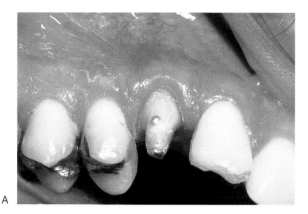

A

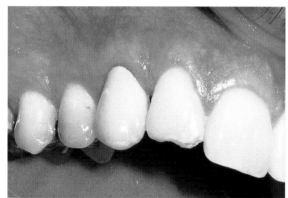

B

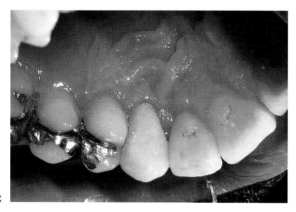

C

Figure 6.26 Patient N after tooth movement had been achieved. (A) Final tooth preparation can be carried out and impressions taken. In this case the Parapost was cemented in place as the final post. Note a little residual Durelay. (B, C) The crown was then completed without compromising aesthetics or the bone support of adjacent teeth.

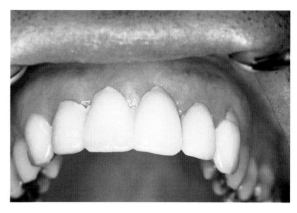

Figure 6.27 Patient O: placement of endosseous dental implants. The patient had damaged both an existing 4-unit bridge replacing the central incisors and the roots of both lateral incisors.

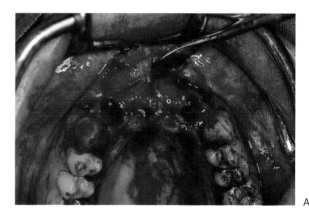

A

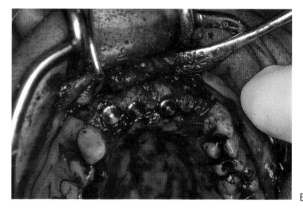

B

Figure 6.28 Prereconstructive placement of implants. The lateral incisors were extracted as atraumatically as possible and implants placed in these sockets as well as in the central incisor sites.

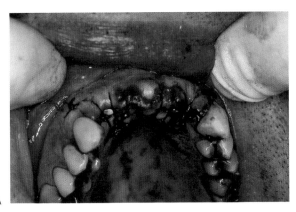

A

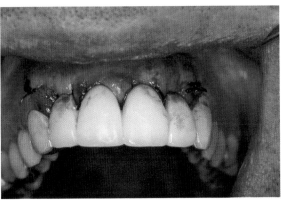

B

Figure 6.29 A temporary resin-retained bridge was bonded in place after the surgical site was sutured closed. Composite pontics were used to facilitate easy adjustment of the pontics in relation to the sutured ridge.

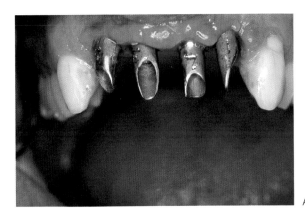

A

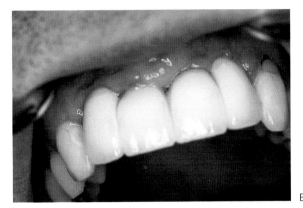

B

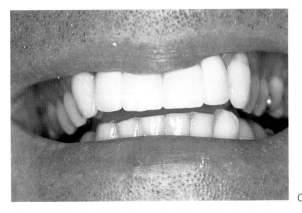

C

Figure 6.30 Patient O: final reconstruction. (A) The implants were integrated and exposed. (B, C) Custom abutments and final implant-supported crowns were made.

before either the dentist or the patient commits to definitive restorations. The philosophy of giving the patient an unattractive temporary restoration, so that they come back for the final, implies a lack of patient education or preparation and is generally an excuse for not taking the time, or having the skills, to make a decent provisional. More importantly, it foregoes the advantage of learning from the provisionals and making necessary modifications before the final restoration is made.

In a treatment planning text, it is inappropriate to go into details of advanced reconstructive care in detail and the reader is referred to standard texts on fixed and removable prosthodontics and implant dentistry. The primary purpose of careful treatment planning and execution is to ensure the smooth completion of this phase in a 'textbook' fashion with a minimum of surprises of complications.

RECALL AND MAINTENANCE CARE

Recall and maintenance involves:

- recall examination
- scale polish and oral prophylaxis
- fluoride application and other preventive measures
- homecare review.

To achieve good long-term care, an effective recall and maintenance programme must be established and executed and it must be customised to the patient's disease susceptibility and specific needs. The concept of a 6-monthly recall for all comes from a toothpaste commercial in the 1940s not from any evidence-based study. While it suits many dentists, and even some insurance companies, to guarantee stable source of income or expenditure with a standard recall period such as every 6 months, it has been questioned and criticised over the years. Lindhe outlined the multiple factors that must be considered in determining a recall frequency and what should go to make up a recall visit. Some patients do need to be seen every 6 months; others are well enough controlled to be seen annually or even less frequently, while considerable evidence exists to justify 3-monthly or even more frequent recall for the most periodontally susceptible as well as patients at high risk of caries.

It is reasonable to inform a patient of the expected recall commitment at the *beginning* of care, not at the end. Patients may think twice about a periodontal treatment plan if advised of the need for 1 hour every 3 months with the hygienist as part of the recall maintenance plan. They should equally be advised of the likely outcomes of inadequate appointment length or frequency. Ultimately, the recall frequency should be agreed between patient and dentist and not dictated by a third party.

7 Business aspects of treatment planning

Most dental practices employ between 3 and 10 staff, operate for around 40 hours a week in premises owned or rented by the owner-manager and derive income by charging a fee for service. These are all classical characteristics of a small business or cottage industry and yet there are those in dentistry who are so focused on the label of a 'profession' that they lose sight of the necessity of applying sound business principles to the management of a general dental practice. While it is beyond the scope of this text to discuss the full spectrum of management in general practice, it is important to consider the various aspects of practice management that impact on treatment planning:

- a rational approach to establishing fees
- establishing ethical payment methods
- appointment control schedules
- the use of appointment control schedules in staff training for effective treatment delivery.

A RATIONAL APPROACH TO ESTABLISHING FEES

At the end of the day, economic principles dictate that, if fees are set too high, patients will not accept them in sufficient numbers to support the viability of the practice, while if they are set too low the dentist will not continue to offer the service in the long run. Between these two extremes, a range exists in which more or less patients will accept treatment, and the dentist will be more or less happy with the fee paid. While it is possible to apply economic theory to establish the elasticity of demand and to calculate an optimum fee for each service offered, in reality a less scientific, more pragmatic approach is generally used.

On many occasions, fees are set by a third party such as the British National Health Service, dental insurance companies or preferred provider organisations. In many countries, regional or national dental associations also provide recommended fee guides that can be used just as references by practitioners but are most often accepted as the 'going rate'.

Rationally, fees should reflect the time taken for a procedure, the fixed and variable overhead costs involved, and the level of complexity and responsibility attached to the procedure. Some consideration should be given to the likelihood of complications occurring within a potential warranty period. Additionally, comparable fees charged by competitors should be considered; however, since there may be no rationality in their development, this may not be a major influence on the final established fee. It is not wise to attempt to differentiate a product based solely on price, and it will be more rewarding if differentiation based on quality of care can be used to justify higher fees.

Historically, laboratory-related types of treatment have been charged at between 2.5 and 4 times the laboratory fees. While this may still be effective in deriving a profit in conventional crown and bridgework, the growth of implant treatment with fairly expensive components purchased from the manufacturer has rendered this formula ineffective. Overall it is best to establish a fee based on the following formula:

time-related costs + variable costs + maintenance/warranty costs
= total fee for procedure

Where *variable costs* are the costs of materials, laboratory-related expenses, component costs, etc., *maintenance/warranty costs* cover a figure built in to cover any likely future problems to be treated gratis, and the *time-related costs* are given by:

(Fixed costs + desired hourly income) × total time spent on procedure

The fixed costs are the hourly costs of rent/mortgage, wages, power, depreciation on equipment, etc. The desired hourly income of the dentist may vary in different areas.

Fixed costs can be established by an accountant. Variable costs can be established based on past experience of similar cases. Maintenance/warranty costs will vary with the level of complexity of the case, the estimated prognosis and the likelihood of a call out. The desired hourly income of the dentist may be consistent for all procedures, but the dentist may wish to place a premium for the most complex procedures where more skill, training and/or responsibility is required. The total time spent on procedure can again be established by reviewing past experience of similar cases.

It is important to remember that few dentists do above average work for below average fees in the long run. A dentist 'forced' to accept low fees by a third party will generally reduce the quality of care by reducing the time spent, the quality of the materials used or the quality of the laboratory selected. When faced with imposed third party fees, the dentist should apply the above formula for each procedure to establish the viability of providing a high quality of care. Clearly the unknown variable to be calculated will be the dentist's hourly rate.

ESTABLISHING ETHICAL PAYMENT METHODS

In the most ideal of all worlds, a dentist should render a service and the patient should pay for the service at the time it is carried out. With the rise in various forms of government and insurance company third party payments, capitation, preferred providers and so on, more complex methods of reimbursement are present in many parts of the world. It is the author's opinion that, whenever possible, the dentist should keep an arm-length relationship with the third party, having the patient pay the dentist directly for treatment and providing basic assistance in securing the reimbursement owing to the patient. This maintains the most direct dentist–patient relationship, keeps the third party in the appropriate place and ensures prompt cash flow for the practice. More importantly, it will instill in the patient a sense of value for the service and potentially a greater sense of responsibility for its maintenance. The more remote the patient is from the financial responsibility for care, the less 'ownership' will exist for the treatment and its long-term maintenance. This is particularly the case when the patient perceives the service as 'free' and knows that any future treatment will also be 'free'. Other than the somewhat intangible prevention of future discomfort, there is

little incentive for patients in this situation to become active, responsible participants in their own care. This has the potential to result in a vicious circle wherein the dentist sees limited effort on the patient's part to look after the dentist's best efforts, and reacts with 'what's the point?', perhaps even unconsciously lowering the standard of care provided.

Clearly it will not always be possible to have the patient pay directly on each visit. Often predetermination of coverage for more advanced procedures and the extent of likely reimbursement is important for the patient in deciding on the choice of treatment, and it may also be a requirement of third party coverage. Patients would clearly prefer to assign the insurance company benefit and only pay any balance due, since this leave them less out of pocket. Insurance companies are likely to prefer one system of bookkeeping, rather than offering several options.

How the dentist approaches the collection of payment due will depend on the regulations involved, the local convention and practice of competitors and, to some degree, the past pattern within the practice. When dealing directly with the patient, the dentist must decide *and clearly communicate to the patient* when payment is expected during treatment. There are several options in use at present.

Payment for each service at the time it is carried out. This not only has the benefit of immediate cash flow but also eliminates the additional costs (stamps, stationery and staff time) involved in sending bills.

Payment at prearranged times within the treatment plan. In extended or complex treatment plans, where many appointments are involved, it is impractical, and perhaps even a little unprofessional, to ask for a payment on each visit. It is equally unrealistic to wait until the end of treatment before a bill is submitted, and so interim payments at clearly prearranged times are preferable. This should be phased to cover large outlays such as laboratory bills and implant component purchases, and it is unwise to have more than 25% outstanding at the completion of treatment. Although bad debts are rare, it is sound business to minimise risk. Equally the dentist and particularly the front office staff should be careful to monitor payment schedules and flag up patients who do not keep to a prearranged schedule.

Payment at the end of treatment. Although, in the past, it has been common for practices to send out bills at the completion of treatment. (I have even come across, within the past 10 years, a practice where some families were billed annually in guineas!) It is not sound business practice to extend such long-term credit. At the very least, monthly statements for amounts outstanding should be rendered. The dentist must be aware that, in effect, the payment when finally received has only a discounted value compared with payment made at the time the service is carried out. The extent of the discount will relate to the waiting period and prevailing rate of interest.

Other payment methods. Some practices, particularly within orthodontics, arrange for a series of *postdated cheques* or *direct debits* to be set up to cover the expected duration of treatment. Others offer a *discount for payment in advance* (usually of around 5%) in extended courses of treatment. Patients will on occasion ask for *extended credit*, with payments extended for several months after treatment is completed. They generally do not expect to pay interest for this credit. Not only does this create significant administrative problems, but it makes little business sense. No bank would extend a loan without building in agreed interest payments. No banker is likely to offer, or agree to carry out, dental treatment as a 'favour' to a client; dentists should not offer or agree to become bankers. When approached along these lines, the dentist can often manage the situation by offering to send the patient's banker a copy of the treatment estimate with a brief covering letter. If banking professionals are then unwilling to extend credit for the proposed treatment, banking amateurs (dentists) would be unwise to take this risk. Again, patients may ask for a discount for cash (black economy)—this is an illegal activity and could result in the loss of the dentist's licence to practice if prosecuted.

In the end, it is for the dentist, working within national ethical and legal expectations, to establish the payment method that best suits the practice. Most important is that the patient is clearly advised of the available methods of payment (cash, credit/debit cards, cheques, etc.), when payments are due and how much is to be paid at agreed times.

APPOINTMENT CONTROL SCHEDULES

Using the principles of sequence of therapy in Chapter 6, it is relatively straightforward to work out the order of treatment to be performed. Even when this has been clearly defined, there are several time-related considerations that come into play:

- necessary time for return of the various stages of laboratory work
- delivery time for special supplies and components not commonly stocked
- healing time after extraction, crown lengthening or other surgery
- maturation time of bone grafts
- tissue improvement time after scaling and root planning
- oral hygiene improvement time needed to show consistent improvement.

When scheduling appointments, it is important that these times are incorporated within the overall treatment schedule. To facilitate this, the author finds an appointment control schedule (Fig. 7.1) an invaluable aid in establishing and maintaining control of the patient's treatment.

This is illustrated in the figure using the example of a patient with the following problems:

- caries to pulp 1-5
- apical abscess 1-5
- caries within biologic width
- desire to keep tooth.

A likely treatment plan may be:

1. Endodontics on 1–5
2. Crown lengthening flap around 1-5
3. Cast post and core
4. Porcelain bonded to gold crown.

Appointments involved would be:

1. Initial endodontics and dressing
2. Complete endodontics and dress
3. Crown-lengthening flap
4. Remove sutures
5. Check healing

	Units	Time Lapse	Procedure	Time	Date
1	3		Initial endodontics and dressing		
		1 week			
2	3		Complete endodontics and dress		
		3 weeks			
3	6		Crown-lengthening flap		
		1 week			
4	1		Remove sutures		
		4 weeks			
5	1		Check healing		
		5 weeks			
6	6		Impressions, post and core, fabricate temporary crown		
		1 week			
7	6		Fit post and core, final crown impression, occlusal records, fabricate temporary crown		
		1 week			
8	2		Cement crown		
9					
10					
11					
12					

Appointment Schedule Dr. _____

Patient _____ H _____

B _____

Figure 7.1 An example of an appointment control schedule with time units of 10 minutes.

6. Impressions, post and core, fabricate temporary crown

7. Fit post and core, final crown impression, occlusal records, fabricate new temporary crown

8. Cement crown.

The time for each appointment should then be determined; for routine procedures this can be preset with front desk or on computer. Most practices work with 10 or 15 minute time units. Once the time units are set for each appointment, and the time lapses between appointments, the appointment schedule can be laid out (Fig. 7.1).

THE USE OF APPOINTMENT CONTROL SCHEDULES IN STAFF TRAINING

It is fundamental to the efficient management of any small business that all of the staff are familiar with the overall mission of the organisation and with their role in achieving that mission. When a patient agrees to the proposals put forward by the dentist and embarks on a sophisticated treatment plan, all of the staff members should be able to interpret clearly what is planned from the patient's records, should have sufficient back-ground knowledge to answer any basic questions asked by the patient and should understand the materials, instruments and other requirements for each visit.

Hence the appointment control schedule, used effectively, should become the 'script' that guides all staff members in delivering efficient care to the patient. By the use of standard procedure designations for each stage, specific tray set-ups should automatically be indicated and should be ready ahead of time (see below). It is beyond the scope of this text to go into details of overall staff training and practice management; however, it should be clear that the appointment control schedule can become an efficient means of communication between dentist, front desk and chairside staff, provided all are familiar with its use. It is also easy to identify times and amount of fees due at specific times within the treatment plan. For the patient schedule given in Figure 7.1, this would be:

Appointment 1: endodontics tray—£100

Appointment 2: endodontics tray—£100

Appointment 3: surgical tray—£300

Appointment 4: postoperative tray—no cost

Appointment 5: examination tray—no cost

Appointment 6: crown and bridge tray—£165

Appointment 7: crown and bridge tray—£250

Appointment 8: crown and bridge tray—£250.

In order to carry treatment to completion, it is important to use the schedule to block book several appointments at the beginning of the sequence and to advise the patient that the appointments are customised to their own plan, are not the same length and, consequently, are not easily interchangeable. This avoids the situation, too often seen in a busy practice, where the next stage can be carried out in 1 week, but the receptionist finds no openings at the patient's preferred time for several weeks.

Practice management has merited several textbooks in its own right, and this chapter has only attempted to highlight the use of sound operations management in the delivery of the patient's treatment plan.

8 Complications and re-treatment

The best laid schemes of mice and men gang aft a-gley

To a mouse, Robert Burns

It is perhaps indicative of the times that consumers no longer expect major purchases to last indefinitely, and that there has been a significant decline in the repair of major appliances in order to extend their useful life. When a microwave, VCR, television or dishwasher breaks down, particularly beyond the warranty period, the owner is as likely to buy a replacement as to seek repair. This is a consequence of both the relatively low purchase costs of the original appliances (usually because of mass production and cheap labour in the second or third world) and the high costs of parts and labour associated with repair in western society.

While it is tempting to consider advanced dentistry in the same vane, there are significant differences. Unlike domestic appliances, initial treatment costs have kept up with or exceeded inflation. Total re-treatment has not only a financial cost but also a time commitment, and a stress and discomfort association. When this is combined with the natural desire of most dentists to do the best job they can, and have it last for as long as possible, we have an obligation to plan complex treatment in such a way that complications are anticipated and, when they develop, are managed in a way that avoids total re-treatment and extends the overall life of the restorations involved. Some dentists will argue against the comparison of advanced dental care with the purchase of domestic appliances, but the business and economics literature clearly identifies the phenomenon of opportunity cost, within which the decision to spend money on a specific item is taken after considering other alternatives on which the funds could be spent. Realistically, the bridge may be postponed because the TV breaks down; the foreign holiday may be cancelled to have the implant this year.

The major difference is that patients expect major dental work to last for a 'long time'. Advice to patients on the realistic life expectancy of different procedures is discussed below and in other chapters. Such figures for life expectancy tend to be based on averages from studies with large sample sizes. The balance of this chapter focuses on the planning of complex treatment in such a way that the longest possible lifespan is achieved, and where possible extended even when complications arise. This involves:

- anticipating complications
- building to the weakest link
- knowing when to patch and when to start afresh.

ANTICIPATING COMPLICATIONS

Until the 1990s, there was little evidence-based research indicating the longevity of the various procedures involved in providing complex treatment to patients. Prior to that, Hirschfeld and Wasserman (1978) and Becker et al. (1979) had shown the long-term efficacy of periodontal therapy; several studies had shown high initial success rates in endodontics and Adell et al. (1981) had shown the long-term success of Branemark titanium implants. Most other areas of general practice had limited if any evidence that could be used to advise patients on the expected longevity of the various aspects of their proposed treatment. Dentists speak of permanent crowns, permanent bridges and permanent cement. As has been previously discussed, this can reasonably be construed, by the patient, to be a guarantee of the permanency of treatment and has been interpreted as such in several jurisdictions.

It is perhaps against the nature of 'perfectionist' dentists to acknowledge that their work will not last forever, but most dentists who have practised in the same location for several years see their failures on a weekly basis. In the last 10 years, numerous publications show expected lifespans for various forms of treatment. In the light of this growing evidence base, it is poor practice to fail to acknowledge the limitations of treatment provided and to fail to plan beyond the life of the work presently being carried out.

It has been my experience that many dentists, including myself, spend the first decade of their career getting into trouble by failing to think long term; the second decade is spent developing innovative ways of getting out of trouble and beyond that comes a point in career development where anticipation and forward planning is more often used to avoid getting into trouble in the first place. While this is often based on personal experience of complications and failures, often associated with unrealistically optimistic treatment planning, it is clearly better to learn from someone else's mistakes than one's own.

There are many simple actions that can turn a potential catastrophic failure, necessitating extensive re-treatment, into a simple maintenance problem. These include:

- use of temporary cement
- design of prosthesis for possible future addition
- the placement of a rest seat for possible future use
- specified undercut or guide plane of a crown, even when a denture is not planned
- planning and noting solder joint placement
- recording of shades
- recording of cements used
- retention of working casts and provisional restorations.

This approach to flexible treatment planning was outlined in detail in Chapter 4.

BUILDING TO THE WEAKEST LINK

It is generally possible, especially in the light of the increasing evidence base, to anticipate which parts of a treatment plan have the highest risk of complications and to plan to manage these when they occur. While several examples of this have been given previously, one of the commonest problems that can occur with bridgework is the wash-out of cement from one abutment while the other remains solid. In time, this leads to caries on the exposed abutment and occlusal trauma on the firm one. In posterior bridgework, the distal abutment is almost always shorted and more tapered than the anterior. A distal wash-out, when the anterior abutment is 'permanently' cemented, can lead to the need to cut off the restoration and complete re-treatment. There are two basic approaches to prevent this major complication: place the whole bridge using temporary cement (acknowledging the risk of loss of retention), or cement the anterior longer abutment with temporary cement and the distal, shorted, sturdier abutment with 'permanent' cement. The second approach often results in long-term retention without problems and, even in the event of anterior wash-out, it is generally straightforward to tap off the bridge distally with little risk of tooth fracture on the molar.

A more elegant, but initially more expensive, approach is to place a telescopic crown on the distal abutment (Fig. 8.1). This is permanently cemented and creates good parallelism with the anterior abutment with minimum taper. The overcase is then cemented using a temporary cement. In the event of distal wash-out, this will occur between metal and metal, negating the risk of caries even if not detected till the next recall.

In some cases, particularly with tooth loss combined with advanced periodontitis, cross-arch splinting is necessary if the life of the remaining teeth is to be extended. In such cases, some movement with possible wash-out is inevitable, and it is often wise to consider telescopic crowns on all the remaining teeth (Fig. 8.2). This approach offers the potential benefit of relatively easy conversion to an overdenture at some point in the future if one or two more teeth are lost. The advent of predictable endosseous implants has reduced the need for this type of management of the terminal decision, but it is still often indicated when an implant option is not feasible.

WHEN TO PATCH AND WHEN TO START AFRESH

Even with careful forward planning, unforeseen complications can occur. Forward planning should allow endodontic complications and porcelain fractures to be managed by removing the restoration, correcting the problem and replacing the restoration. Caries is the commonest complication, which, by compromising marginal fit of the restoration, may present the dilemma of deciding between a patch and a total re-treatment. When considering patching a cast restoration that has developed caries, the operator should consider several questions.

Apart from the caries, is the restoration intact? It is impossible to use radiographs to determine the extent of the caries. If the crown or bridge can be removed, the extent of caries will be clear;

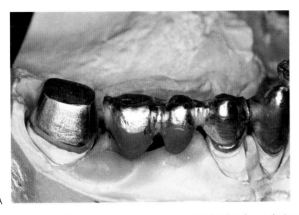
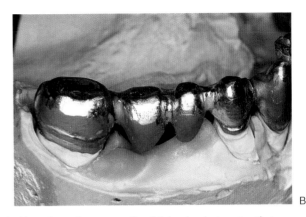

A
B

Figure 8.1 This long span lower posterior bridge has been designed with a telescopic crown on the distal molar abutment so that cement wash-out, if it occurs, will most likely occur between the telescope (cemented with permanent cement) and overcase (cemented with temporary cement). Note that the distal embrasure will be a soldered joint while the anterior embrasures are cast joints. This allows for the strongest framework if the molar is ever lost and conversion to a cantilever becomes necessary.

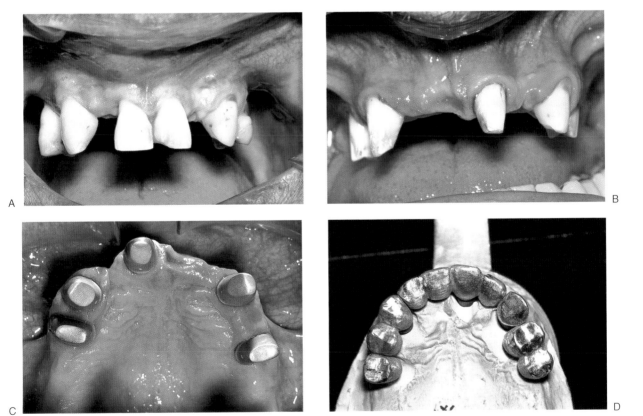

A
B

C
D

Figure 8.2 This patient has advanced periodontitis complicated by tooth loss and significant mobility. He is not coping well with a partial denture and wishes to consider a fixed restorative option. For health reasons implants are not a practical option. (A) Before treatment. (B) One incisor has been lost and the remaining teeth are prepared for full crowns. (C) Telescopic crowns with a parallel path of insertion are fabricated and will eventually be cemented with a permanent cement. (D) A one-piece fixed bridge overcase is fabricated with a single cantilever unit on the left side. (This is consistent with the shortened dental arch concept described in Ch. 4.)

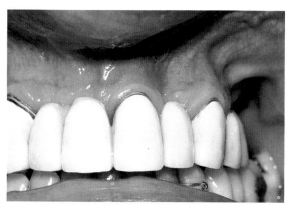

E

Figure 8.2, cont'd (E) The final prosthesis is completed using acrylic resin rather than porcelain. This is because the potential mobility of the bridge as a whole may lead to porcelain fracture, and the cross-arch stability of a single section is essential to extend the life of the remaining teeth. Composite resin is also a potential veneering material.

however, if the problem is with one abutment on an extensive bridge, it is essential to try to establish if there is also cement wash-out, because if a patch filling is placed in such a situation, not only will it fail but additional caries may progress undetected until pulpal involvement occurs.

Is the pulp still healthy? If a patch filling is followed by the development of endodontic problems on the tooth, and the need for an access preparation through the occlusal or palatal, the total loss of tooth structure is likely to result in loss of cement retention and secondary caries. While pulp testing is difficult on a crowned tooth, it is usually feasible by a combination of thermal and radiographic tests to determine the state of the pulp. If still in doubt, caries removal should proceed carefully without anaesthetic, using a slow

speed round bur. This will give the same information as a test cavity.

Will patching compromise future re-treatment? If removal of caries will create a significant undercut, which may compromise a future crown, then it is wiser to consider total re-treatment initially rather than merely patching the tooth.

Will the patch compromise the retention of the crown? Any caries removal around the margin of a crown will, to some extent, reduce the retention of the original restoration. The clinician must determine, as far as is feasible, the extent to which retention will be compromised, and the likely outcome of this. Clearly if the original dies have been retained, the dentist is in a much better position to assess the likely results of reduced retention.

How long has the restoration been in place? While this should not override the above clinical considerations, it is wise, when such a problem develops within a year or two of original placement, to consider the goodwill created by full re-treatment as against the potential ill-will created by patching. The situation is clearly different when the restoration has been placed elsewhere, and here advice should be based on clinical findings alone.

What does the patient want? Last, but certainly not least, are the patient's wishes on how the situation should be managed. The dentist's role is to provide options with the benefits and disadvantages of each, and the patient must then reach an informed decision. Where a compromise is forced on the dentist, the patient must accept a greater amount of responsibility for the outcome, as was the case outlined when compromise treatment plans were discussed in Chapter 4.

9

Treatment planning: medico-legal issues

John A.D. Cameron

INTRODUCTION

When a dentist provides dental care or treatment for a patient, the dentist has a *duty of care* toward that patient to provide them with safe, effective dental care, of a standard an individual patient has a right to expect from a practitioner holding themselves to be skilled in that particular discipline. By providing a patient with a treatment plan, a dentist is, in effect, making an offer to a patient; in many instances, the treatment plan will provide the basis for a *contract* between the dentist and the patient. Furthermore, the treatment will be fundamental in the process of obtaining a valid *consent*; treatment carried out without consent may be trespass, battery and/or assault, and treatment without consent could in certain circumstances lead to criminal conviction.

NEGLIGENCE: THE DUTY OF CARE

The law establishing a duty of care

In order to establish that, in law, a dentist has a duty of care toward a patient, it is not necessary to go back as far as the leading negligence case of Donoghue v. Stevenson (1932 AC 562) when it was established that the manufacturer of a bottle of ginger beer owed a duty of care to people who might drink its contents. The law makes it quite clear that anyone who holds him or herself out as being prepared to give dental advice or treatment impliedly undertakes that they possess the necessary skill and knowledge that a dentist is expected to have. Not only that, a dentist who is consulted by a patient owes that patient a duty of care when deciding whether to undertake the case, a duty of care when deciding what is the appropriate treatment, a duty of care when carrying out that treatment and a duty of care in answering any question from the patient when the dentist is or should be aware that the patient intends to rely on the answer. A breach of

This chapter is by John A. D. Cameron, Dental Adviser, The Medical and Dental Defence Union of Scotland.

any of these duties could give rise to an allegation of a failure to exercise one's duty of care and a possible claim of negligence (Bolam v. Friern Hospital Management Committee (1957), All ER 118; [1957] 1 WLR 582).

The degree of skill the law requires

A dentist must practice with a reasonable degree of skill and knowledge, exercising a reasonable degree of care, being aware that failure to use due skill in diagnosis resulting in inappropriate treatment is in itself negligence. Dentists are not required to have the highest or lowest levels of care, skill and competence, each individual case is judged on its own merits; that is what is required by law. If a practitioner of greater skill or knowledge would have prescribed different treatment or executed it differently, that is not indicative of negligence, nor is it negligence if a dentist has acted in accordance with a practice accepted as proper by a responsible body of dentists, even though a body of adverse opinion also exists among dental practitioners. Furthermore, a dentist can act in accordance with one responsible body of dental opinion in preference to another in relation to the diagnosis and treatment without being negligent, provided that that particular practice is reasonable.

Variations in treatment

Additionally, the law does permit dentists to carry out forms of treatment others might not, because in order to establish liability for negligence on that basis, *it must be* shown that there is a usual and normal practice, that the practitioner has not adopted it and the treatment carried out is such that no professional person of ordinary skill would have proceeded in that way if he or she had been acting with ordinary care (Clark v. MacLennan (1983) 1 All ER 416).

Skill and experience

However, it is imperative that dentists are aware that, although the duty of care required in law is that of a reasonable and careful practitioner of the same grade or level of experience (Wilsher v. Essex Area Health Authority (1987) QB 730 [1986] 3 All ER 801 CA), inexperience is no defence; an inexperienced practitioner would be expected to seek help or guidance from an experienced practitioner (Wilsher v. Essex Area Health Authority, 1987); failure to do so is a failure in their duty of care to the patient.

Accepting referrals

Senior colleagues should be aware of their responsibility to give appropriate advice in accordance with their duty of care when consulted by juniors, including a further referral to a more suitably qualified or experienced colleague if it would be inappropriate, given their skill and experience in the particular matter, to give the advice requested personally.

Failure to exercise one's duty of care

Any patient who feels that their dental care has fallen below the standard that they believe they have a right to expect may raise an action against their dentist, citing negligence due to a failure by the practitioner to exercise their duty of care appropriately. In order to resist any such action or allegation, a dentist should be mindful of the fact that expert evidence will be required to support this assertion by their patient, but also they themselves will require to produce expert opinion to uphold that their advice, diagnosis, treatment planning and treatment was that of a dentist exercising *reasonable* skill. Although a patient alleging negligence may be examined by the experts, the main body of evidence available to a dentist to resist such a claim will be contained within their clinical records, practice protocols and information supplied to the patient.

Expert evidence

Experts relied upon should be of a similar standing within the profession to the dentist complained against. The standard expected of a general dental practitioner should be that afforded by a body of reasonable general dental practitioners and not the standards of a specialist. Similarly, someone offering themselves to patients or colleagues as a specialist in a particular dental discipline would be expected to exhibit the skills of a body of specialists in that same discipline.

DENTAL CARE IN RELATION TO THE LAW REGARDING CONTRACT

The nature of a contract

A contract is an agreement, enforceable by law, the intention of the parties being to create legal relations. A contract may be written or verbal and may have expressed as well as implied terms. For a contract to be binding, it must be freely entered into (i.e. without threat), include an offer and an acceptance as well as a *consideration*, which in the dentist's case will usually be in the form of payment to the dentist. The expressed terms within a contract will be those contained within the contract as part of the offer, such as the provision of specific treatment or availability to provide care and treatment. Implied terms of the contract will be those such as, 'treatment will be appropriate and carried out with reasonable skill'. A breach of a condition within a contract may well give rights to either party to terminate that contract. Dentists should also be aware that contractual liability is generally strict (that is fault or lack of it is irrelevant—it is no use stating, 'I wasn't to blame'); it may be argued that strict liability does not apply to the service element, where the dentist must carry out diagnosis, treatment planning and treatment with reasonable skill and care, but that is debatable.

Third party funding

Dental treatment may be paid for directly by the patient, indirectly by the patient through a third party or directly by a third party such as an insurer, government or health authority. Third party funding either directly or indirectly involves contracts being entered into by the dentist, the third party funder and the patient; these are often extremely complex and dentists should ensure that both they and their patients fully understand the precise nature of the contracts that they are entering into, as well as the rights and obligations they place upon them all. Third party funders frequently have clauses within their contracts requiring dentists to undertake treatment according to specific rules, to keep available records containing particular information, or to fulfil certain requirements regarding premises and equipment. Dentists should not disregard these contractual obligations before entering into such a contract or during its duration.

Contracts with patients

Treatment plans will often be the basis of an offer to a patient by a dentist to provide that patient contractually with goods and/or services; the plans must, therefore, be carefully written to ensure that the dentist can reasonably fulfil the offer being made both in the expressed and implied terms of the contract. Practitioners must also be aware that any remarks made to a patient during diagnosis and treatment planning inferring or stating a result, such as 'You will be able to eat better', 'Your family will be sure to think you look better' or 'This restoration will last 20 years', may well be construed as implied or expressed terms of the contract if a patient subsequently raises an action for breach of contract.

Government funding

In jurisdictions where governments fund dental care, there may, in fact, be no contract between the patient and the dentist even though the patient pays the majority of the fees through statutory charges. Dentists often consider that the contractual requirements between the dentist and the funding government body place seemingly onerous unnecessary conditions upon a practitioner in order to make claims. These terms should not be disregarded nor treated with disdain; in law, making a claim for payment, thereby inferring that one is complying with the conditions necessary to make that claim, might well lead to an accusation that the dentist has made a false statement to gain financially knowing that such a claim was invalid. This could result in criminal charges, and even imprisonment, if the dentist is found guilty.

Legislation

All countries within the European Union (EU) have consumer laws. In the UK, the most frequently cited is the Sale of Goods Act 1979; in relation to dentures. However, other consumer protection legislation may well apply to dentistry, such as the Supply of Goods and Services Act 1982, the Consumer Protection Act 1987, or even the Consumer Credit Act 1974, where dentists are supplying goods or services by way of credit facilities. Furthermore, the method in which a particular government enacts legislation may well permit a form of dental treatment in one jurisdiction but forbid it in another. (The UK incorporated an EU

directive defining cosmetics into UK legislation that made it an offence to use 'named products for bleaching teeth' in the UK, although their use was permitted in other EU countries.)

CONSENT

The meaning of consent

Consent may be implied; this would occur if a patient rang a surgery requesting an appointment for a dental check-up, came into the surgery, sat in the chair and was examined by the dentist. However, implied consent should never be assumed without the practitioner being absolutely sure of the nature of the patient's attendance and having regard to the fact that any implied consent will be highly specific, such as only for a visual examination, not a radiograph. In general, dental practice consent is normally given verbally, the dentist informing the patient of the proposed treatment and the patient giving verbal approval. *Written consent* is not frequently obtained by general dental practitioners but must be obtained for general anaesthetics and sedation; the prudent would also obtain it for complex, particularly irreversible, treatment plans, as well as for treatments carrying a significant risk according to the literature, such as extractions of lower third molars or other oral surgery procedures.

The consenting process

The legal age

The first requirement in the consenting process is to establish the competency of the patient to give their consent to any procedure, which includes diagnosis and treatment planning. The legal age for consent varies in different jurisdictions, and practitioners must be aware of the legal requirements in the territories in which they work. Generally speaking, irrespective of age, young people below the age of majority may well be able to consent to dental treatment as long as they are able to understand the nature of that treatment, the consequences of that treatment and the risks involved, as well as having the ability to comprehend the alternatives and make a reasoned decision (Gillick v. West Norfolk and Wisbech Health Authority (1985) 3 WLR 830, CA). Dentists should also be aware that in England and Wales the Children's Act 1989 prevents children below the age of 18 refusing treatment if their appropriate parent(s) consent on their behalf. However, this would appear to be a legal anomaly, given that the selfsame child, if adjudged competent, can agree to have the treatment but not apparently withdraw that consent as an adult can. Consenting by adults above the legal age for consent still requires a determination that the patient is competent, but this is generally easily facilitated other than in the handicapped. Dentists must be aware that consent can be withdrawn at any time, and no one adjudged competent can be forced to have treatment against their will.

Adults with incapacity

In the majority of jurisdictions, no adult can consent on behalf of another adult; therefore if an adult is incompetent in relation to themselves, a consenting process must be gone through to obtain as much information as possible. The practitioner must come to a decision based on the 'best interest test' as to what treatment, in the circumstances is in the best interests of the patient, mindful that the rationale chosen must be capable of being deemed appropriate by a body of reasonable practitioners. Although individual circumstances will require differing requirements as to how much knowledge can or should be obtained, agreed written protocols would appear to be the best way to ensure compliance with the law and employers' stipulations in this respect.

The treatment

Consent is required both for the treatment and the method by which the treatment is to be delivered. If treatment is to be carried out using some form of physical restraint, relative analgesia, sedation or general anaesthetic, then consent is required for that additionally. Furthermore, both with regard to treatment and method of delivery, a patient cannot consent unless they are given sufficient information regarding the alternatives and the risks to come to an informed decision. Establishing what information is required to be given will depend upon the circumstances, but again this will need to be capable of withstanding scrutiny and be in accord with what would be considered reasonable by a body of reasonable practitioners. Although patients should be given *sufficient* information to consent, explicit information regarding surgical technique may not be necessary where this might unreasonably frighten the patient; it would similarly appear inappropriate to inform patients of complications that rarely happen and are unlikely to happen in the circumstances.

Written consent

Written consents should contain details of all the information given to the patient to enable them to come to their decision giving consent, particularly with regard to treatment alternatives, risks and costs. Patients are entitled to receive an itemised account for treatment where this is appropriate and requested. Consent is dynamic; competency may vary according to the treatment to be undertaken and the method of delivery, as well as with the age or mental capacity of the patient. However, any specific requirements of the patient with regard to eating, drinking, operating moving machinery or looking after dependants subsequent to treatment must be made clear to the patient and included on the consent form. It would seem to be good practice for both the patient and the dentist to retain copies of any written consent.

RESISTING CLAIMS

Risk management

Adequate treatment planning is essential even for the simplest dental intervention. The prudent dentist would be well advised not only to have strict protocols and guidelines for treatment planning and treatment but also to be able to demonstrate to anyone reviewing a particular case that his or her treatment planning and treatment was carried out with an appropriate degree of skill and attention. An agitated patient, or a judge, will rely upon an expert to examine all the available evidence and come to a decision on whether there has been a failure in the dentist's duty of care, a breach of contract, or a failure to comply with consumer legislation or gain a valid consent. Invariably, the best opportunity to resist a claim is by having comprehensive information available within the dentist's records and clinical notes.

The role of the expert

Patients have a right to a 'basic' standard of care; courts, patients and their legal teams often rely on experts who are academic dentists working in dental teaching hospitals. Although not general practitioners, they are often more adept at writing reports than practitioners and will have ready access to the dental literature to support their opinions. They will generally have postgraduate qualifications and, in litigious jurisdictions, will likely be more conversant with the legal process than the practitioner, having been asked for their opinions on a number of occasions. They will likely be distinguished within their chosen field and may be skilful in the witness box.

Dental records

As many claims against dentists occur long after the event, it is vital that dentists keep and retain full, accurate, contemporaneous dental records that reflect the patient's condition and their complaint at each and every consultation. The records must contain full details of the diagnosis, advice given, treatment carried out, treatment alternatives, options and warnings that were given at each and every appointment. Figure 9.1 shows an example treatment record. It is particularly pertinent that records are capable of demonstrating treatment efficacy and how patients' teeth and their gums respond to treatment over a period of time. Computerised and written clinical dental records should be capable of producing a chart or audit trail showing teeth and gums sequentially. No matter which notation is used to record teeth, it should be clear to patients and dentist alike. The use of the dental cruciate with teeth noted apparently transposed left to

right on the page is confusing to non-dentists. Treatment plans and reports given to patients or lay people should record teeth as per their position *in the patient's head* (i.e. upper left 7 or upper left second molar), informing patients with a diagram if deemed appropriate.

Retention of records

The length of time that records must be retained varies from jurisdiction to jurisdiction; the absolute minimum should be 8 years after the last attendance or 8 years after the patient attains the age of majority. Practitioners should be aware that some third party funders may only require record retention for a period much shorter than that which might be required in law. As a general rule, records should be retained for as long as possible because, in the majority of jurisdictions, patients can raise actions a number of years after they become aware of the problem giving rise to the claim, which might, by definition, be an indefinite period thereafter. In some countries within the EU, there are statutory legal requirements as to what is required to be recorded on patients' dental records, and dentists practising in

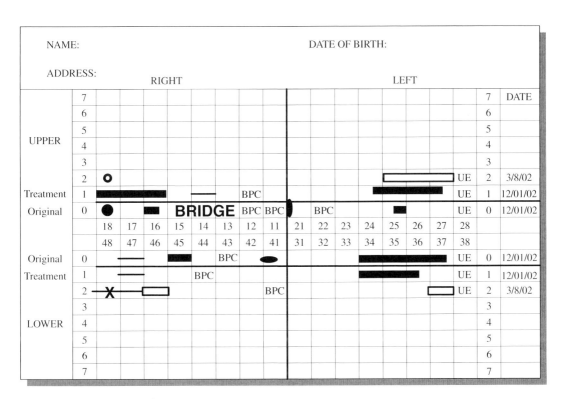

Figure 9.1 A treatment record.

these jurisdictions must be aware of these requirements. Even where specific notation is not a requirement by statute, it is frequently a requirement of third party funders, indemnifiers and insurers; consequently, dentists should comply if they do not wish to jeopardise their rights to payment of fees or indemnity.

Medical history record

Any patient seeking treatment or advice from a dentist should have a comprehensive medical history taken; findings must be recorded and the history updated, recording that the updating has taken place prior to any subsequent surgical or dental intervention. The relevance of a comprehensive and full medical history will depend upon the treatment envisaged, but it must be established that patients have not only fully understood all the questions but also their relevance to the treatment that they are about to receive, and replied appropriately. Dentists should ensure that any 'medical alerts' cannot be missed by being placed obscurely in the record; visual or audible alerts are useful with computerised records. Computerised records must be 'password protected' and written records safeguarded to maintain confidentiality. It is useful to record on the front of dental record cards, the dates that medical histories have been updated and any changes noted (Fig. 9.2).

General clinical records

With the exception of those only wishing emergency care, most patients expect to receive ongoing care and advice to enable them to maintain their dentitions for as long as possible. It is essential, therefore, that a dentist can exhibit that he or she has monitored oral health over the years, carried out the necessary tests, given the appropriate advice and carried out suitable treatment to address problems as and when they arise,

including, if possible, advice regarding preventing problems in an effort to sustain the patient's dentition. All warnings, alternative possible diagnoses and treatment plans should be recorded. In order to provide evidence that such monitoring has taken place, it is, therefore, necessary to have a 'baseline' condition report for the first visit of a patient to the surgery. This should include a full soft tissue, periodontal tissue and hard tissue examination with full recording. The subsequent records should present a serial view of the individual's ongoing oral health tooth by tooth and area by area. This will support the view to any observer that the patient has received appropriate ongoing care and treatment.

Periodontal record

Periodontal chartings must be evident, as well as oral hygiene, dietary advice, toothbrush instruction, etc. Full periodontal chartings will be necessary on occasions, particularly when complex, advanced courses of treatment are to be undertaken, coding such as CPITN (Community Periodontal Index of Treatment Needs) or BPE (Basic Periodontal Examination) on others. Caries and periodontal disease should normally be controlled prior to embarking on advanced courses of treatment; this cannot be ascertained without proper record. Failure by the patient to comply with instructions or advice given must be recorded, including appointments when the patient failed to attend. Any expert perusing the records must be able to elicit that dental decay, periodontal problems and any other oral disease have been correctly recognised, diagnosed and treated, if the patient has consented; any refusal to accept treatment or advice must similarly be noted.

Record of treatment required

In addition to the baseline full charting, a note of all the missing teeth, restorations present, restorations defective as well as the teeth requiring attention should be evident. Periodontal tissues should be assessed and periodontal treatment and its outcome should be noted as well as any recommendations for equipment necessary to assist cleaning and with ongoing caries experience. Patients' dental histories should be vigorously assessed and recorded with relevant personal habits/conditions. Tests such as percussion, vitality, trans-illumination, thermal tests, pathology, when carried out, should be noted and commented upon both to necessity and result within the record. Patients' treatment plans should be confirmed within

NAME:				DATE OF BIRTH:	
ADDRESS:					
MEDICAL HISTORY					
Date	Change	Date	Change	Date	Change

Figure 9.2 Update of medical history.

the notes, as should differential diagnoses, alternative treatment plans, warnings, potential difficulties, intended outcomes, etc. If treatment is subsequently changed, the reasons for variation from what was originally planned should be noted along with problems encountered. It should also be evident from the record why one particular treatment plan rather than another was undertaken. Copies of treatment plans given to patients should be retained.

Record of radiographs, tests and models

A radiographic assessment of disease risk and the time interval considered appropriate for radiographs such as bitewings should be made for all patients other than those seeking casual treatment. This should be recorded on the record along with a notation of the next due date, with the reason for any due date being varied. The necessity for radiographs, photographs and any other tests should be thoroughly assessed (Fig. 9.3). Radiographs should be taken according to assessed clinical needs, the practitioner being mindful of the benefits and shortcomings of each type of radiograph. Beam locators should be used; radiography resisted by the patient should be recorded. Conventional radiographs should be mounted, named and dated; these and any radiological examination must be commented upon and retained within the body of the record, including reasons for their exposure. Digitalised radiographs should be saved in a format demonstrating that they have not been, and cannot be, altered. Clinical photographs provide graphic information to patients as well as recording the necessity for treatment, disease progress and the incidence of marks, artefacts, discoloured teeth, etc. not readily recordable in any other format. Any pathological tests, their necessity and outcome must be recorded as well

NAME: DATE OF BIRTH:

ADDRESS:

RADIOGRAPHIC ASSESSMENT REGARDING CARIES AND PERIODONTAL DISEASE

Risk assessment: Interval for bitewing:

Next BWS		Next BWS	

Figure 9.3 Example of radiographic assessment and monitoring.

as copies of referral letters and responses received. Study models are an adjunct to good diagnosis and treatment planning; their value should never be underestimated.

Records of treatment delivery

Great care should also be taken to record the mechanism by which treatment is intended to be delivered for an individual patient, particularly regarding patients with special needs. If restraint in the form of physical restraint, conscious sedation or general anaesthesia is to be used, the reasons for this must be noted and the appropriate consent obtained. If a particular treatment regimen is to be undertaken because of difficulties in delivery or the patient's inability to maintain good oral hygiene, rather than the treatment that might be considered by another as the preferred option, this should be noted in the clinical record.

Referral of patients

A dentist has an ethical obligation to assess the treatment required and refer the patient for specialist help or a second opinion if they are unable to come to a diagnosis, the treatment is beyond their expertise or the patient requests such a second opinion. Patients are demanding and dentistry is a difficult task; dentists must ensure that they are never pressurised into carrying out treatment that is unwise, of dubious value or against their better judgment. Care should be taken, particularly when restoring teeth of doubtful prognosis at the patient's behest, that the potential benefits outweigh the risks.

Consent

The records must demonstrate that a consenting process has be undertaken and a valid consent from a competent individual obtained in all but exceptional circumstances. Many claims allege that consent for the treatment had not been properly obtained, patients stressing that if they had been aware of the process or the outcome they would not have agreed to the treatment being carried out, remonstrating that it had not been fully explained, despite the practitioner's protestations to the contrary. Dentists must hone and audit their communication skills, doing all that they can to ensure patients comprehend what they are told. Without adequate records and explanations contained within the dental record, as well as a written treatment plan, an allegation of failing to obtain proper consent is sometimes difficult to resist. An allegation of trespass due to lack of consent does not require proof of *causation* (harm or loss resulting) as is required to be successful in negligence. Patients should be advised of treatment plans even in simplest cases, using written plans in the more complex; practitioners must resist the temptation to use jargon when describing treatment.

Addressing the patient's problems

The practitioner's duty of care to a patient extends to addressing the problems that they attend reporting; a wise precaution to resist claims, particularly of continued pain, would be for dentists to ensure that they record negative as well as positive findings everytime a patient attends. It will prove invaluable to counteract many allegations if the first entry after the date states what is the patient's complaint, recording even when there is no complaint. When a patient attends with a problem, it is incumbent upon the dentist to deal with that problem, so this must be clearly evident from the notes, particularly if the decision is taken that no intervention is required. Reviews, denture eases, matters under observation and any matters still to be addressed or to be dealt with at subsequent appointments must be recorded.

Indemnity

Every dentist should carry adequate indemnity or insurance to protect and recompense patients in the event that they make an error of judgment or a mistake during treatment. Patients do have a right to expect dentists to be competent; they also have a right to expect recompense when things go wrong as a result of some error, mismanagement or misjudgment by the practitioner. Dentists must comply with the regulatory authorities, employers and contract holders regarding registration, postgraduate education, cross-infection control, etc.

CONCLUSION

Hindsight

Hindsight is a wonderful educator but can be a cold bedfellow in times of trouble. Peer review and clinical audit of treatment and treatment outcomes are essen-

tial tools, along with continued professional development, to demonstrate that dentists have taken adequate steps to ensure that their treatment planning and treatment outcomes are contemporary, appropriate and in the patient's best interests.

Learning from our mistakes

Whenever a mistake occurs, particularly if it could be described as an 'untoward incident', it should be carefully analysed, lessons learnt and the whole matter comprehensively recorded. Admitting fallibility rather than displaying arrogance may well be the best tool, along with comprehensive records, to prevent a simple error of judgment becoming a catastrophe. The contents of this book reflect the art and science of sound treatment planning; however, that treatment planning cannot be adjudged as sound if there is no evidence to support such a judgment in any retrospective analysis. Written protocols and guidelines are essential; if a dentist diverges from what is regarded as *usual*, that decision must be justified and reflected in the clinical record. Dentists should be as equally proud of their dental records as they are of their clinical work. Lecturers generally show their slides, hoping to receive praise and admiration; less frequently do we see open exhibits of their disasters—that is human nature. We can all marvel and admire the artistry of the competent clinician; we should also be able to admire and marvel at the artistry of the competent clinician's clinical records and their ability to learn from their mistakes.

Avoiding stress

Dentistry is hard work, physically and mentally, it is extremely stressful; by having and following guidance, protocols and accepted sound clinical standards within one's own practice, together with maintaining accurate comprehensive contemporaneous records, one reason for stress should be considerably reduced. Let there be no mistake, claims or the threat of claims together with complaints are upsetting and harrowing; we must all have the ammunition readily available to justify what we have done, not only for the protection of our patients but more especially for the protection of ourselves and our own peace of mind.

10 Treatment planning in aesthetic dentistry

While there has always been an aesthetic component to general dental practice, the period since the early 1980s has seen a huge increase both in the range of aesthetic services offered to patients and the aesthetic demands and expectations of patients. The improvements in bonding technology, the evolution of veneers and other improved ceramics, the rise in professional and self-application bleaching methods, the growth in cosmetic periodontal surgery and many other advances have led to an aesthetic revolution for which many dentists have not been well prepared in dental school.

New materials and techniques will continue to be introduced; however, basic principles of developing a pleasing cosmetic result are, like basic occlusal principles, likely to stand the test of time. It is appropriate to review these basic aesthetics principles here, since they have a major impact on the treatment planning of a patient whose chief complaint is of an aesthetic nature. The chapter then attempts to take the basic principles of treatment planning outlined in previous chapters and to apply them, using general aesthetic guidelines, to the rapidly growing area of aesthetic dentistry.

FUNDAMENTAL AESTHETIC PRINCIPLES

The endpoint of effective aesthetic dentistry is for the dentist to create a result that registers with the viewer as being 'an attractive smile', without drawing attention to itself. The viewer should take in the smile, at an unconscious level, register its attractiveness, but then return to the patient's eyes to continue conversation. Realistically, a good result should stand scrutiny from 4 feet (1.2 metres) away in conversation. It is unrealistic to expect any artificial material to simulate nature when scrutinised from 6 inches (15 centimetres) away, with lip retractors in place or when projected onto a screen. A patient who has to pull their lips up to let you see their 'chief aesthetic complaint' should only be approached with great care, if accepted for treatment at all.

Key to effective aesthetic treatment planning is the identification of what concerns the patient about the appearance of their teeth. Since aesthetic procedures are, by their nature, elective, it is crucial that the dentist clearly establishes what the patient is looking for and then assesses the feasibility of providing it. Historically, we have not been well trained in assessing aesthetic problems, and some patients, while aware that they do not like the look of their teeth, find it hard to express exactly what is wrong. In making an assessment, three factors must be considered.

- proportion (the golden proportion)
- symmetry
- harmony.

The golden proportion

Much has been written about the relationship between height and width, known as the golden proportion. This ratio of 1.6:1 appears to transcend cultural differences and is found around the world both in architecture and art; it represents a ratio that is universally considered pleasing.

Dentally, the golden proportion is seen in the ratio of height to width of the incisor teeth, and in the relative width of central and lateral incisors. In the context of the face, it is repeated in the ratio of width from the outer aspects of the eyes in relation to the eye to mouth distance.

The closer aesthetic dentistry comes to maintaining or creating the golden proportion, the more pleasing the results are likely to be. Much of the basis of planning aesthetic care involves recognising variances from this ratio and planning its establishment. The danger in merely applying the techniques available is that the dentist will be so focused on good impressions and accurate margins, that 'the big picture' can be missed. While it is easily technically possible to close a diastema, if this results in a gross violation of the golden proportion, it is not likely to be well received.

Symmetry

Much of what is pleasing in a smile is the relative symmetry of left and right sides. Again, the greater the variance from this, the less pleasing the smile is likely to be. Treatment planning for aesthetic improvement should be based on moving towards the most symmetric result possible. Three aspects of symmetry should be considered:

- width
- height
- depth.

Width

Width is by far the most important dimension when attempting to achieve aesthetic symmetry. Even with a relatively low smile line, the incisal half of the teeth will likely be visible and a lack of width symmetry will be noted in most patients (Fig. 10.1). For this patient, there was a discrepancy in the widths between the central and lateral incisors and a radical form of treatment was needed to restore symmetry. After several diagnostic wax ups, it was felt that width symmetry could only be achieved by extraction of the right incisors and major orthodontics or by extraction of all incisors and fabrication of an implant-supported or tooth-supported bridge. The patient had hoped that crowns alone could improve the situation and treatment was declined.

Height

Height is the next most important dimension. While variations in incisal length will again be noticeable with all smile lines, variations in the gingival margin will only be noticed with a relatively high smile line. Hence ridge augmentations and gingival margin realignments should not be recommended to patients with low smile lines. Patients who seek this probably have unrealistic aesthetic demands, and dentists who offer it should ask themselves what is the real rationale for treatment. Figure 10.2 shows a patient with a low smile line where height asymmetry of the incisal edges has been corrected by simple cosmetic recontouring. No consideration of gingival margins is needed. Figure 10.3 shows another patient with a height variation between canines at the gingival margins. The right canine has erupted bucally, resulting in considerable variation in height. Because of the high smile line, the

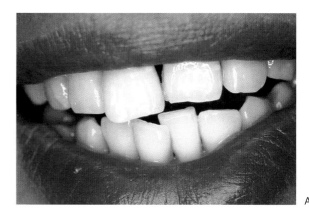

A

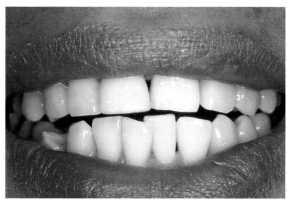

B

Figure 10.1 An extreme example of an aesthetic problem caused by a discrepancy in the widths between central and lateral incisors. Here a radical form of treatment may be needed to restore symmetry.

Figure 10.2 (A) A 36-year-old female with aesthetic concerns about the uneven lengths of her incisors. (B) Since she had a low smile line, simple aesthetic recontouring in the incisal edges was sufficient to manage her aesthetic concerns.

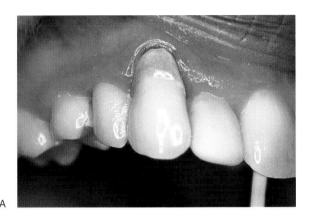

A

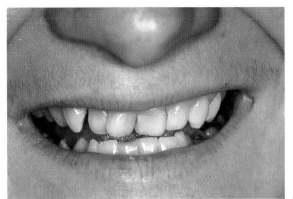

A

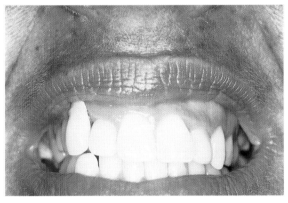

B

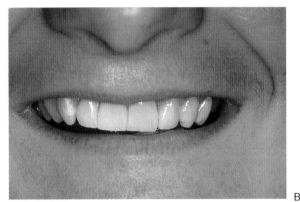

B

Figure 10.3 A 34-year-old female who has complained of the appearance of her right canine. (A) The right canine has erupted bucally. (B) This resulting variation in the gingival height of the canines is very apparent because of her high smile line.

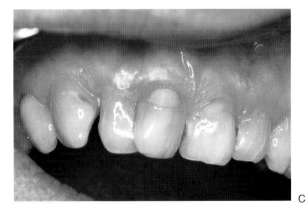

C

Figure 10.4 Improving the aesthetic situation for a woman with significant anterior crowding. (A) Before treatment. (B) After treatment with veneers of varying thickness, which appear symmetrical from the anterior view. (C) The right central incisor is overlapped onto the lateral incisor. *Continued*

height variation in symmetry is very apparent and significant; relatively complex treatment would be necessary to manage such a problem. It is apparent that the previous crowning and use of pink porcelain has been unsatisfactory in correcting the aesthetic problem. Ideally, comprehensive orthondontics or at least localised eruption of the tooth followed by a new restoration would be needed to manage this height asymmetry problem. It is essential here to consider both soft and hard tissue, and treatment becomes more complex.

Depth

Depth is by far the least noticed dimension. Our sense of depth is much less astute than that for width or height: we only have to think how difficult it is to identify a class 2 division 1 malocclusion when viewed from the front. This relatively poor depth perception can often be used to advantage. Figure 10.4A shows the before and 10.4B the after smile view of a 39-year-old patient with significant anterior crowding who has had veneers of varying thickness. While width symmetry could not be achieved without orthodontics, the illusion of symmetry was created by taking advantage of

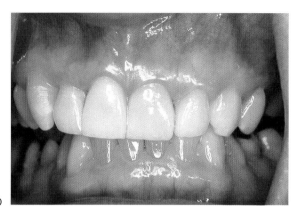

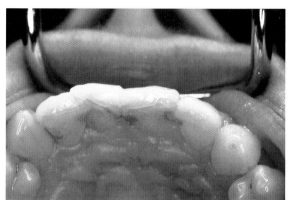

D   E

Figure 10.4, cont'd (D) The lateral incisor is overlapped onto the canine. (E) When viewed from below, the overlapping and actual lack of symmetry becomes very apparent.

our relatively poor depth perception. Also note that, as the patient is happier with her smile, the right side of the lip goes higher and reveals more tooth (Fig. 10.4B). By overlapping the right central incisor onto the lateral and the lateral onto the canine, the illusion of symmetry could be created in the four incisors. This is achieved in part by the psychological phenomenon of *closure*, whereby, in the appropriate context, a viewer seeing part of a familiar shape will subconsciously register the whole shape (Fig. 10.4C,D).

Harmony

Harmony is a more subjective assessment than symmetry. With regard to dental aesthetics, it generally relates to the relationship of hard to soft tissues: the harmony of the incisal edges with the lower lip and the harmony of the gingival margins both with each other and with the upper lip.

Smile line aesthetics

In recent years the term *smile line aesthetics* has entered the dental literature. This refers to the assessment of the overall appearance of the teeth and gums when the patient smiles. The basic classifications of smile lines can be broken down into four types.

- *low smile line*: less than 50% of incisal height of the upper anterior teeth, and no gingival margin is visible in a natural full smile (Fig. 10.5). In this type of smile line, width symmetry is the important feature.

- *medium smile line*: between 50 and 100% of the incisal height of the upper anterior teeth, and the

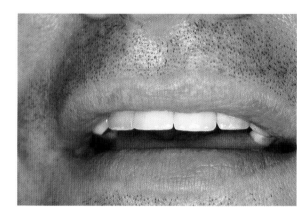

Figure 10.5 A low smile line. Less than 50% of incisal height of the upper anterior teeth and no gingiva is visible in a natural full smile. Since the visible parts are symmetrical, the effect is pleasing.

papillae are visible in a natural full smile. The marginal gingivae is, however, not visible (Fig. 10.6). Again width symmetry is the important feature, although height may also be relevant if loss of papillae occurs.

- *high smile line*: all of the height of the upper anterior teeth as well as all of the papillae and marginal gingivae are visible in a natural full smile (Fig 10.7). Both width and height are important and soft tissue position and symmetry must always be considered.

- *gummy smile*: all of the height of the upper anterior teeth as well as an excessive amount of soft tissue is visible (Fig. 10.8).

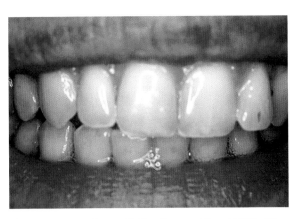

Figure 10.6 A medium smile line. Between 50 and 100% of the incisal height of the upper anterior teeth and the papillae are visible in a natural full smile.

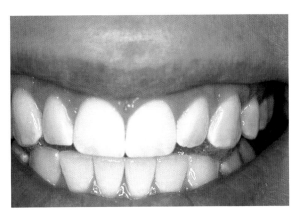

Figure 10.9 Bone recontouring via an apically positioned flap corrected the width to height ratio in the patient shown in Figure 10.8 to closer to the golden proportion. Excessive gingival tissue was also removed.

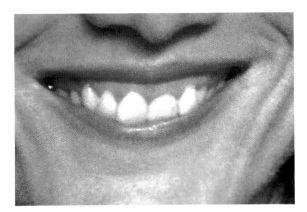

Figure 10.7 A high smile line with all of the height of the upper anterior teeth as well as all of the papillae and marginal gingivae visible in a natural full smile.

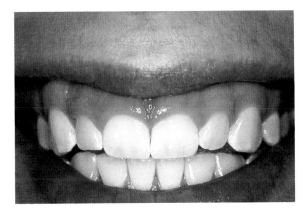

Figure 10.8 A gummy smile with all of the height of the upper anterior teeth as well as an excessive amount of soft tissue visible.

The patient with a gummy smile, shown in Figure 10.8, had just completed over 2 years of fixed orthodontics and was disappointed with the overall result; this was the major active problem in her mouth. The width to height ratio of incisors was closer to 1:1 than to the golden proportion and a diagnosis of delayed passive eruption was made. Bone recontouring via an apically positioned flap corrected the width to height ratio to closer to the golden proportion; excessive visible gingival tissue was also repositioned (Fig. 10.9). More importantly, the patient was then happy.

Most patients would appear to be seeking both symmetry and a medium-to-high smile line. We must bear in mind however that with the ageing process, and the progressive loss of collagen tone combined with gravity, the lips progressively droop as the patient ages. Hence the high smile line in a 20 year old will not generally look either natural or pleasing in a 70 year old. Beware the pensioner who brings the smiles from Vogue or Elle when trying to explain their wishes (Fig. 10.10). The 73-year-old patient shown in Figure 10.10 had recently had a reconstruction with upper anterior crowns. She felt that something was 'not right' but admitted that she took several fashion magazines to her previous dentist to show him the smile she wanted. The height to width ratio is too great and much too much tooth is visible for the patient's age.

Altered (delayed) passive eruption

The majority of gummy smiles are the result of some form of delayed passive eruption (Fig. 10.8). While

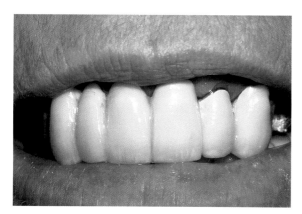

Figure 10.10 A 73-year-old woman who has had upper anterior crowns that have resulted in too great a height to width ratio for her age.

Coslet et al. (1977) offer a complex classification of this condition, it is sufficient to recognise three classic features:

- the gingiva is higher on the crown of the tooth than normal for the patient's age
- the appearance is generally of square teeth; not fulfilling the golden proportion
- bone *may* extend onto enamel.

Although Coslet et al. offer a subclass of delayed passive eruption where only the soft tissue stays abnormally high, this cannot be easily diagnosed either clinically or radiographically.

If surgical management is contemplated, then a flap procedure with an initial internal bevel incision is always safer, since it allows an initial visualisation of the buccal bone height before a decision is made on the necessity for bone as well as soft tissue removal (Fig. 10.9). A conventional gingivectomy with no visualisation of bone can lead to tissue removal close to bone, and an inevitable re-growth and failure to maintain the desired cosmetic result.

Gingival aesthetics

With regards to gingival aesthetics, certain features are generally considered pleasing:

- gingival symmetry: the left and right sides should be close to mirror images of each other
- harmony between tooth and gum visible: neither a toothy nor a gummy smile is present; the 'ideal' harmony is referred to as the 'gull wing' appearance

- pontics that appear to 'grow' from tissue
- no black triangles.

The 'gull wing' appearance

The gull wing appearance is made up of:

- bilateral symmetry
- a gingival margin on the upper that drops from central to lateral incisor then rises from lateral incisor to canine resulting in visible gingivae of
  —0.5 to 1 mm above the central incisor
  —1.5 to 2 mm above the lateral incisor
  —0 to 0.5 mm above the canine.

The gingival rise and fall should be in harmony with the upper lip line, while the incisal edges of the six anterior teeth should have a similar 'gull wing' rise and fall, which again harmonises with the lower lip.

Pontics 'growing from tissue'

More traditional methods of extracting teeth has often led to the destruction of the remaining buccal plate, with resulting aesthetic defects in patients with high smile lines. The resulting ridge defect often forces the dentist to place an unaesthetic pontic that is longer gingivally than the contralateral tooth and which often stands out from the ridge, throwing a shadow on the tissue (Fig. 10.11A).

Black triangles

The loss of the interproximal papilla, resulting in a 'black triangle', can be a devastating aesthetic problem in a patient with a high or even medium smile line. This problem is greatest between upper central incisors but can affect all anterior papillae to some extent. Since the surgical rebuilding of an interdental papilla is at best unpredictable, every effort should be made to preserve the papilla where it is present. Where a defect is present, it can, on occasion, be reduced by a combination of periodontal, restorative and even orthodontic procedures.

PROCEDURES TO IMPROVE SYMMETRY AND ACHIEVE A PLEASING COSMETIC RESULT

Procedures that can be used to improve aesthetic appearances include:

- periodontal plastic surgery
- orthodontic procedures

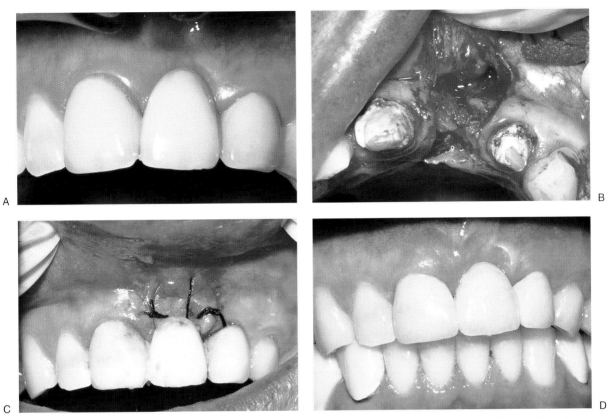

A   B   C   D

Figure 10.11 An old bridge replacing the left central incisor has a ridge lap pontic over a ridge with considerable loss of buccal plate. (A) This results in asymmetry due to a long pontic, shadowing and a generally false-looking tooth. (B) An envelope flap is taken back and connective tissue graft placed to augment the buccal deficiency. (C) The pontic is recontoured and shortened and the site is sutured. (D) After a period of healing, the new bridge is made, using an ovate type of pontic. Now the pontic appears to grow out of the tissue and better symmetry has been established.

- restorative procedures
- combined approaches.

Periodontal plastic surgery

Ridge augmentation

Figures 10.11 and 10.12 illustrate soft tissue augmentation procedures where the primary objectives are to replace tissue lost through trauma, resorption or infection. The aesthetic objective is to create the illusion of the pontics growing out of the tissue rather than sitting on top of it and to move the aesthetics towards a symmetrical appearance.

Ridge reduction

Ridge reduction is used where extraction has resulted in loss of papillae architecture between the replacement teeth. A gingivoplasty procedure is used to recreate

the illusion of papillae and to allow more pontic space to achieve the proper height to width ratio (Fig. 10.13).

Recession correction by grafting

Figure 10.14 illustrates the use of connective tissue grafting to correct recession and restore symmetry.

Crown-lengthening flap surgery

Crown-lengthening flap surgery can be undertaken for symmetry and/or harmony and/or proportion. Figure 10.15 shows the change achieved when a gummy smile is managed by an apically positioned flap in a young female model. This 17-year-old model was concerned about the appearance of her front teeth. Initially she requested veneers to improve the appearance. The problem was diagnosed as delayed passive eruption, resulting in both a gummy smile and poor width to height ratio of anterior teeth. After healing, a pleasing

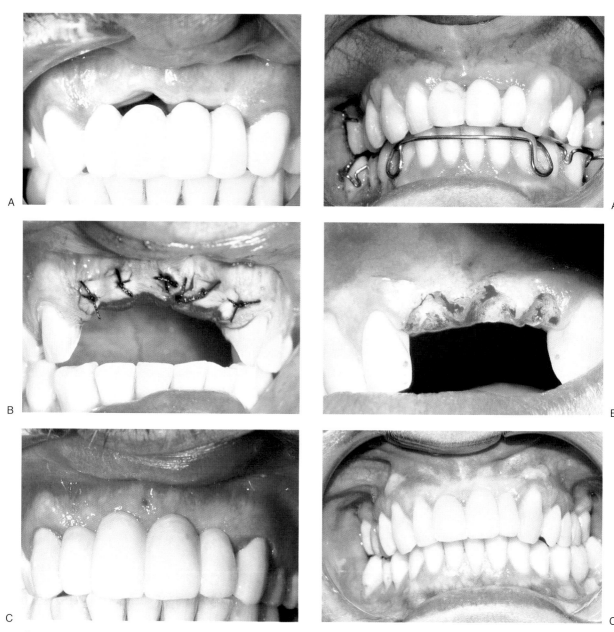

A

B

C

A

B

C

Figure 10.12 A major height deficiency in the ridge is present owing to traumatic loss of teeth and considerable alveolus. (A) The provisional bridge has been prepared on a model with the ridge waxed back to the desired contour as a guide to the surgeon. (B) An onlay graft type of ridge augmentation procedure has been carried out to restore some ridge height. (C) After healing the final bridge is made and symmetry restored by a combination in soft tissue augmentation and porcelain extension.

Figure 10.13 Ridge reduction. (A) Many years in a partial denture has resulted in flattening of the ridge with loss of definition of the papillae. (B) After needle probing to confirm adequate tissue thickness, a gingivoplasty procedure was carried out to redefine the papillae and establish sufficient space for longer pontics. An immediate reline of the denture guides tissue healing. (C) A resin-retained bridge has now been made, again incorporating ovate pontics and re-establishing a better symmetry between incisors. Note how much closer the final result is to a gull wing appearance and golden proportion than in (A).

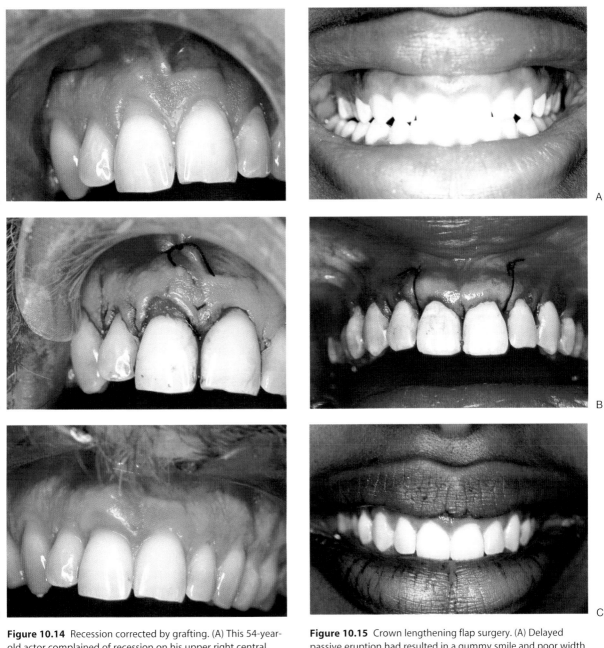

Figure 10.14 Recession corrected by grafting. (A) This 54-year-old actor complained of recession on his upper right central incisor. (B) A connective tissue graft was placed using the technique described by Langer and Langer (1986). Blood supply come from the underside of the flap and the periostium. (C) After healing, the recession has been corrected and symmetry restored.

Figure 10.15 Crown lengthening flap surgery. (A) Delayed passive eruption had resulted in a gummy smile and poor width to height ratio for the anterior teeth. (B) An apically positioned flap with ostectomy was carried out, moving tissue to a position agreed with the patient on study models. (C) After healing.

gull wing appearance was achieved, the width to height ratio was improved and the patient was delighted. Most importantly, this result was achieved without any irreversible treatment of the teeth.

Orthodontic procedures

Space regaining and diastema closure

The 23-year-old patient shown in Figure 10.16 presented with major asymmetry caused by a congenitally missing lateral incisor and a peg lateral. There was also evidence of parafunction and of spacing in the anterior teeth. Significant fixed orthodontics was needed to reposition the teeth, close the diastema and reopen the pontic space for final symmetrical restorations (Fig. 10.16B).

Eruption of soft tissue

The technique of forced eruption, originally described by Ingber in the 1970s for improvement of bony defects, can be adapted for the movement of gingival margins where significant asymmetry is present and crown lengthening is contraindicated. Figure 10.17 shows a 19-year-old female who had fractured her right central incisor in a biking accident. The fracture was supra-gingival on the palatal but ran 4 mm subgingival on the buccal in addition to the significant recession and loss of buccal plate. The situation was complicated by a high smile line. Her general dentist has root treated the tooth and placed a temporary crown. After considering all options, it was decided to erupt the right central incisor in order to bring down the gingival

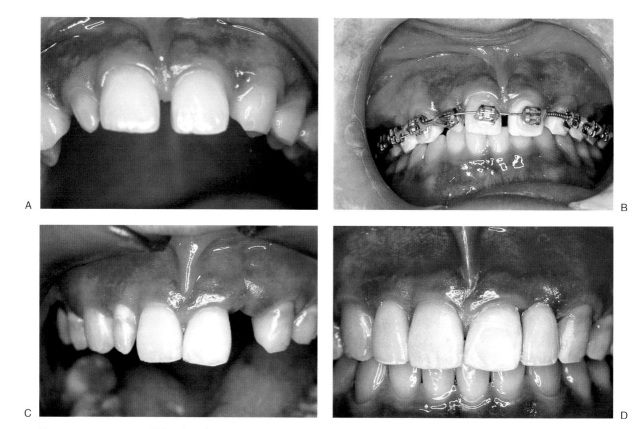

A

B

C

D

Figure 10.16 A 23-year-old female with major asymmetry caused by a congenitally missing lateral incisor and a peg lateral, as well as spacing between anterior teeth. (A) Her appearance was causing her significant concern. (B) After acceptance of a diagnostic wax up, localised orthodontics was initiated to reposition the teeth, close the diastemas and reopen the pontic space for final symmetrical restorations. (C) Tooth movement and subsequent crown lengthening has been completed. The surgery has not only exposed all of the natural enamel, moving closer to the golden proportion, but has also, palatally, exposed the maximum amount of enamel area for bonding of the planned resin-retained bridge. (D) Final restorations consist of a double-winged resin-retained bridge replacing the left lateral incisor and a porcelain veneer on the right lateral incisor. Compare the symmetry with the appearance at presentation and note the gull wing appearance and gingival and incisal margins.

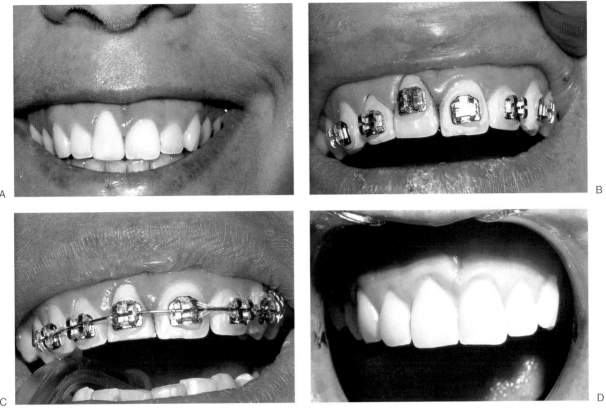

Figure 10.17 Forced eruption to move gingival margins. (A) A right central incisor fracture with significant recession and loss of buccal plate was complicated by the high smile line. The incisor had been root treated and fitted with a temporary crown. (B) The right central incisor was forced to erupt. (C) Tooth movement has brought down the gingival margin; the erupting tooth was kept out of occlusion. (D) After tooth movement was completed, a limited ostectomy moved the biological width beyond the fracture line and reduced the gummy smile. After healing, a final crown was completed.

margin to match the other central incisor. The patient was advised that the tooth would be slightly narrower at the gingival level but that this could likely be masked restoratively. Tooth movement progressively brought down the gingival margin and on each visit, the occlusion was checked and the erupting tooth taken out of occlusion. After completion of tooth movement, an apically positioned flap with limited ostectomy was carried out to reduce the gummy smile and move the biological width beyond the fracture line on the right central incisor. A healing period of at least 16 weeks is generally advised, and the final crown was then made for the right central incisor.

Restorative procedures

Restorative procedures include veneers, cosmetic contouring, crowns, bridges and implants. These have all been discussed previously.

Combined management

It is most important for the dentist to realise that there is no single panacea that will correct all aesthetic problems. It is best to be familiar with all of the available procedures, to diagnose the patient's presenting problems accurately, differentiating between hard and soft tissue factors, and then to develop a treatment plan to address these problems using the appropriate procedures. Most commonly, a combination of procedures is necessary to achieve the best overall result. For the patients illustrated in Figures 10.16 and 10.17, periodontal flap surgery was also an integral part of achieving the overall result.

Adapting treatment planning principles to new technologies

Never be the first to take up a new method, nor the last to abandon an old one

Sir William Osler, physician 1849–1919.

WHEN IS A NEW TECHNOLOGY STILL EXPERIMENTAL?

Dentists historically have been slow in adopting new technologies. The high-speed drill was largely developed in the 1940s but did not become widely used until the 1960s. Bonacore developed acid etching and the basics of adhesive dentistry in the 1950s and again it was 20 years before these advances reached practice. Branemark treated the first of his implant patients in 1965 and published long-term data in 1981, thus converting implant dentistry from an 'art' to a 'science'; yet, even today, not all dentists offer implants as a treatment option. Guided tissue regeneration was conceived by Melcher in 1971 and is still considered as *new* by many dentists.

On the other extreme, some dentists love new 'toys' and are anxious to be seen to be up to date and present this image to their patients. While it is hard for a patient to differentiate between the leading edge and the lunatic fringe, this should not be the case for the health professional. Too often in the past, we have been influenced by the oratory skills of a dynamic speaker, rather than the data presented. This situation is often nurtured by some manufacturers and laboratories in order to reach a critical sales volume for their equipment and products. Many areas of dentistry have been exposed to this aggressive marketing of unproven 'aids'. Over the last few years, several 'periodontal susceptibility' tests have been marketed that use methods perhaps of interest to the research scientist but certainly of no proven clinical value. Dyes to detect precancerous oral lesions have caused considerable debate. Practices advertise as offering 'laser dentistry' or 'no-drill fillings' while the associated techniques have at best limited application in general practice. 'Mercury-free' practices abound

while substantiating literature is lacking and the patient is often the loser in terms of quality of care as well as expenditure.

Between the two extremes lies the middle ground where most good dentistry is practiced. New techniques should be constantly assessed but only adopted if they offer a benefit over the established alternative (see evidence-based dentistry, below). It is simplistic to suggest that one technique or piece of equipment can replace many others. Sound advice, offered many years ago is 'Never join a society which worships one technique or piece of equipment'. We cannot conceive of a 'Society of high-speed drill dentistry' or an 'International Association of Retraction Cord Users' yet we are asked to join societies built around lasers, electrosurgery or gold foil. For the same reason, it is unlikely and undesirable that dental specialities should develop around single techniques. The desire to have a speciality of implantology is too narrowly technique focused to be practical. Implantology is a fundamental part of several disciplines rather than a speciality in isolation.

As new techniques evolve, their evidence base must be assessed; when proven adequate, the techniques can find a place within general practice that is still applying basic sound principles of treatment planning, occlusion and so on. Generally the practising dentist should look for at least two independent multi-centred studies, blind or double blind where feasible, and of at least 3 and preferably 5 years' duration, before considering offering a new technique or material to patients. Universities and laboratories, with appropriate consent, are the proper place for research into new materials, not the mouth of a general practice patient.

EVIDENCE-BASED DENTISTRY

Too often in the past the main influence on change in general practice was the sales representative from a dental supply company or the charismatic speaker, often sponsored by one company to present their products in a favourable light. Dental students have historically taken the word of their lecturers and textbooks and have had little if any experience in objectively reviewing the literature. While this may have produced fairly effective technicians, it leaves dentists with limited training in appraising new products or techniques.

Ultimately, we will be held accountable for our actions by what is published in the dental literature and not what a lecturer or salesperson told us, and it is essential for the modern dentist to be able to apply the principles of evidence-based dentistry on a daily basis, but particularly when evaluating a new product or technique. It is beyond the remit of this book to expand on the principles of evidence-based dentistry, and the reader is referred to several excellent articles and texts on the subject.

IMPACT OF DENTAL IMPLANTS

Although their full potential is not yet appreciated by all dentists, the advent of predictable dental implants, largely based on the work of Branemark, has totally revolutionised dental treatment planning.

In the descriptions of patients treated with various combinations of implants that follow, the reader should stop and look at each, asking one simple question, 'How would this patient have been treated before implants?'

Figure 11.1 shows a 16-year-old girl who, without implants, would be condemned to partial dentures for the rest of her life, a victim not of dental neglect but of the biological anomaly of congenitally missing teeth. Limited orthodontics and orthognathic surgery was carried out to reduce the open bite and improve tooth

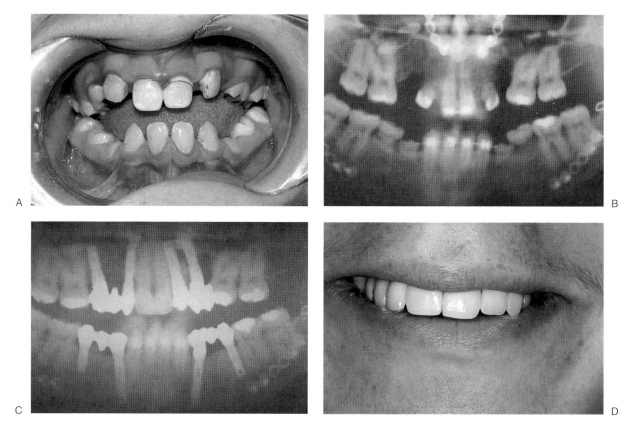

Figure 11.1 A 16-year-old girl with multiple retained deciduous teeth, congenitally missing permanent teeth as well as an anterior open bite. (A) Initial appearance. (B) Orthopantomogram shows the missing teeth and retained deciduous teeth. (C) Eight implants support 12 units of implant-supported bridgework. (D) Veneers have been placed on the central incisors.

position. The use of implants to support bridgework (Fig. 11.1d) has restored the patient to a satisfactory aesthetic and functional situation without the need for partial dentures. Without implants, the patient would be condemned to a lifetime of partial dentures. The final result is an intact dentition that is aesthetically pleasing and functionally sound.

The 18-year-old girl in Figure 11.2 presented with the challenge of a missing canine with virgin teeth with large pulps as potential abutments. In this situation, neither one tooth partial dentures or resin-retained bridges are likely to do well; to cut down adjacent teeth

for full-crown abutments has a high risk of endodontic complication, has a limited lifespan and is, of course, totally irreversible. The implant-supported crown is, in fact, the only relatively long-term fixed restoration for this situation. The final restoration was aesthetically acceptable and involved no damage to tooth structure or linkage to adjacent teeth, with the associated risks and oral hygiene complications. A shallow group function has been established. Normal orthodontic retention was followed. The adjacent teeth have not been involved in the restoration and this restoration offers the best long-term prognosis of all alternatives.

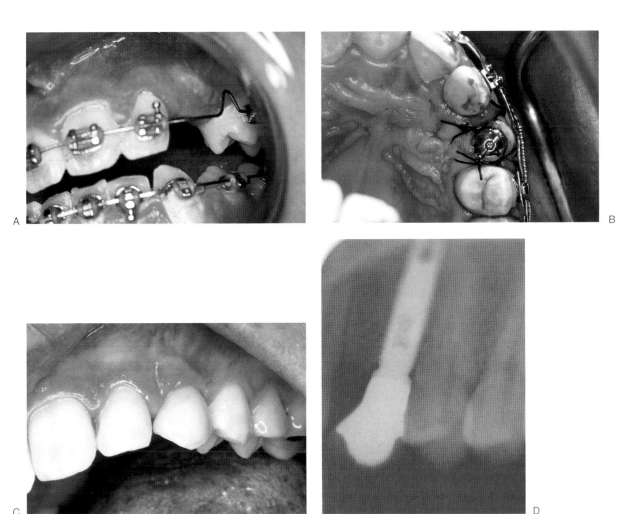

Figure 11.2 Replacement of a missing canine tooth. (A) This 18-year-old has had an impacted canine tooth removed and is coming close to completion of orthodontics. (B) Implant placement was carried out just prior to final anterior retraction. This allowed the implant surgeon a little more space and meant that the implant exposure and completion of orthodontics closely coincided. (C) The final restoration, which is aesthetically acceptable and involves no adjacent teeth. (D) The final radiograph shows a well-integrated 15 mm implant adjacent to two healthy natural teeth.

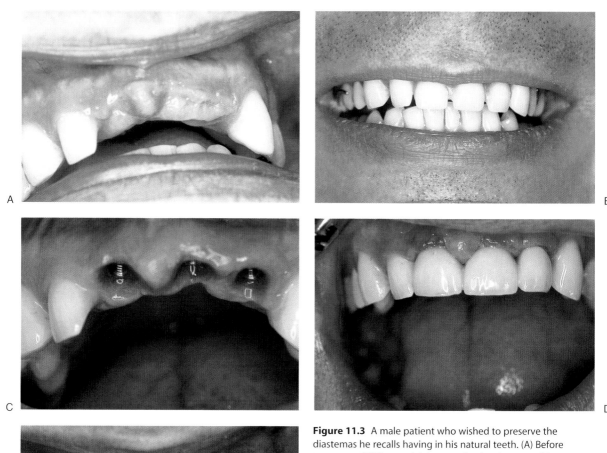

Figure 11.3 A male patient who wished to preserve the diastemas he recalls having in his natural teeth. (A) Before treatment. (B) The partial denture that has been used for many years, which reproduces the diastemas. (C) Implants were placed trying to preserve what papillae contour remains and to allow tooth support in an agreed position retaining diastemas. (D) As a final confirmation, the provisional crowns were initially made connected with all diastemas closed. This confirmed his desire to retain spacing. Aesthetics are poor because of the poor width to height ratio. (E) The final implant-supported crowns restored the original diastemas.

Figures 11.3 shows a businessman who has worn an upper partial denture for many years. His own incisors had natural diastemas and he has rejected fixed bridgework in the past since the diastemas could not be included, and he wished to avoid cutting down healthy teeth. Single implant-supported crowns offer a predictable way of recreating the original diastemas while eliminating the partial denture. To confirm that the patient was certain of his wish to preserve diastemas, an initial provisional bridge was made with the teeth linked (Fig. 11.3D). It should be noted that the width to height ratio of incisors here was unfavourable (see Ch. 10). This confirmed the superior aesthetics of retaining the diastemas, and the case was completed as the patient wished. Although bridgework was feasible for this patient, it could not address the patient's aesthetic wishes and would be destructive of tooth structure.

The 62-year-old university researcher shown in Figure 11.4 had also worn a partial denture for several years to restore a seven tooth edentulous span and a single missing left premolar. He made a quality of life decision to eliminate the denture and replace the missing teeth with implants. Apart from the denture and implant-supported restorations, there were no other treatment options for this situation. The long-term prognosis of implant restorations is excellent and in this patient the use of implants has removed any additional loading from the remaining teeth, thus improving their prognosis.

FUTURE EFFECTS OF IMPLANT TECHNOLOGY

When realisation of the full potential of implants reaches the majority of general practices, several

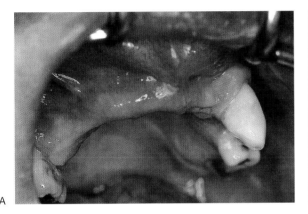

A

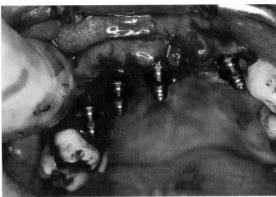

B

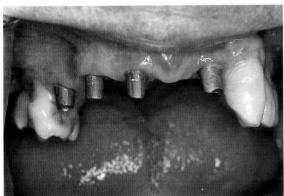

C

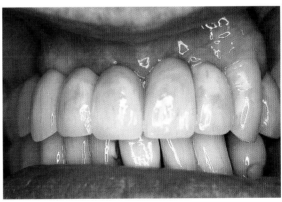

D

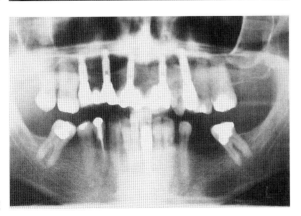

E

Figure 11.4 Elimination of the need for a partial denture. (A) The patient had a seven tooth edentulous span and a single missing left premolar. (B) A total of five titanium implants ranging from 13 to 15 mm in length were placed in the maxilla. (C) After successful integration and healing, custom abutments were fabricated on the implants. (D) The final porcelain bonded to gold alloy implant-supported bridge and single crown were fabricated, custom shaded and inserted with temporary cement. All embrasure spaces were checked for oral hygiene access with floss threaders or interproximal brushes. (E) The final radiograph shows excellent support for the implant bridge.

significant changes in practice patterns will occur, all of which will have a major impact on treatment planning.

Complete dentures will no longer be the end of the line. Even when a patient looks to be heading towards a complete denture, the dentist should be thinking beyond the denture and should take no action that will reduce the opportunity to go on later to implants if necessary. This will necessitate more attention being paid to bone preservation during extractions.

Extractions will alter to improve bone preservation. Extractions will be slower and more carefully carried out, with a focus on bone preservation and possible augmentation with bone grafting and/or guided bone regeneration. Extraction by tooth rotation and expansion to the buccal, followed after the tooth has been removed by compression of the socket was perhaps appropriate in the 19th and part of the 20th century; however, as this can lead to narrowing of the ridge and a buccal aesthetic defect, it is not appropriate in the 21st century.

Some teeth will be taken out sooner. If we know we are going to lose a battle we should focus on winning the war. Since implant success rates are higher with longer implants, and since implants have been shown to assist in bone preservation, it makes sense to extract teeth with very poor prognoses while some bone remains as a potential foundation for future implants.

More strategic extractions will take place. Often a few remaining teeth occupy a position where implants would ideally be placed. In order to achieve an optimum result, these teeth may be sacrificed although they may have survived for several more years.

The use of long-term partial dentures will decline. As implants are more widely used, the partial denture will often only be used as an interim restoration until implants can be placed. While there will always be a role for the partial denture as a compromise restoration, its use as a definitive solution to an edentulous situation will be significantly reduced.

Fewer teeth will be cut down as bridge abutments. While resin-retained bridges have, over the past few years, offered more conservative medium-term options for small edentulous spaces, the combina-

tion of declining caries rates and the implant option will dramatically reduce the number of full crown abutments for fixed bridges. Although most dentists take it for granted that it is reasonable to cut down two adjacent teeth to support a fixed tooth replacement, imagine the trauma if you were a lawyer or accountant rather than a dentist: you have just lost a treasured upper anterior tooth and the 'solution' is to cut down two adjacent teeth. This mindset will have to change rapidly. Even today, dentists consider the fixed bridge to be the 'conventional' restoration, when in fact the implant has a better evidence base, better long-term prognosis and is more conservative of the remaining dentition.

As a proven technique, the use of dental implants should be a consideration whenever any form of tooth replacement is being considered within a treatment plan. While not always appropriate or indicated, they are often the treatment of choice and as such dentists have a moral and ethical obligation to offer them to appropriate patients. All dentists must pause before cutting down relatively healthy abutment teeth and ask themselves if this irreversible step is really the treatment of choice and in the patient's best interests. Dentists should ask themselves how they would treat a family member with the same problem. If the dentists plans to treat the patient in the chair any differently, ask why.

While some dental schools already give the undergraduate student limited exposure to implant dentistry, the discussion of their indications and contraindications must really become a fundamental part of the teaching of treatment planning as well as restorative dentistry. It is much more appropriate for the dental student to be given a solid, evidence-based generic grounding in the subject than to be exposed to implants for the first time in a company-sponsored weekend hotel course.

Dental implants are used as an illustration of a 'new' technique that has evolved from a non-evidence-based art in the 1950s and 1960s, through a university tested method in the 1970s, into a soundly established method of treating partial and total edentulism since the 1980s.

While the advent of evidence-based osseointegrated dental implants has had a major impact on the options within, and details of, treatment planning in general practice, it does not in any way alter the principles outlined in the preceding chapters.

References and further reading

Abrams L 1980 Augmentation of the deformed residual edentulous ridge. Compendium, 205–214

Adell R, Lekholm U, Rockler B, Branemark PI 1981 A 15 year study of osseointegrated implants in the treatment of the edentulous jaw. Int J Oral Surg 10, 387

Ainamo J, Barmes D, Beagrie G, Cutress T, Martin J 1982 Development of the World Health Organization Community Periodontal Index of Treatment Needs (CPITN). Int Dent J 32, 281

Amsterdam M 1974 Periodontal prosthesis 25 years in retrospect. Alpha Omegan, December, 9–52

Aukes JN, Kayser AF, Felling JA 1988 The subjective experience of mastication in subjects with shortened dental arches. J Oral Rehab, 15, 321–324

Becker W, Berg L, Becker EB 1979 Untreated periodontal disease; a longitudinal study. J Periodontol 50, 234–244

Coslet JG, Vanarsdall RL, Weisgold A 1977 Diagnosis and classification of delayed passive eruption. Alpha Omegan 10, 24

Garber D, Salama M 1996 The aesthetic smile: diagnosis and treatment. Periodontology 2000, 11: 18–28

Goldstein RE 1982 Change your smile. Quintessence Publishing, Atlanta, GA

Hirschfeld L, Wasserman B 1978 A long term survey of tooth loss in 600 treated periodontal patients. J Periodontol 49, 229

Ingber JS 1974 Forced eruption 1. J Periodontol 45: 199

Ingber JS 1976 Forced eruption 2. J Periodontol 47: 203

Ingber JS 1989 Forced eruption; alteration of soft tissue cosmetic deformities. Int J Perio Rest Dent 9, 417

Ingber JS, Rose LF, Coslet JG 1977 The biologic width; a concept in periodontics and restorative dentistry. Alpha Omegan 10, 62

Kayser AF 1981 Shortened dental arches and oral function. J Oral Rehab, 8, 457–462

Kayser AF 1994 Limited treatment goals: shortened dental arches. Periodontology 4, 7–14

Kois J 1996 The restorative-periodontal interface: biologic parameters. Periodontology 2000, 11: 29–38

Langer B, Langer L 1986 Subepithelial graft technique for root coverage. J Periodontol 55, 715

McCarthy FM 1972 Emergencies in Dental Practice, 2nd edn. Saunders, Philadelphia, PA

Okesan JP 1985 Fundamentals of occlusion and temporomandibular disorders. Mosby. St Louis. MO

Tarnow D, Eskow R, Zamzok J 1996 Aesthetics and implant dentistry. Periodontology 2000, 11: 85–94

Appendix

LONG MEDICAL HISTORY

The Dental Specialists' Group

Name _____ Date of Birth _____ Marital Status _____
      Last   First   Middle   Day M. Yr.

Address _____ Phone _____

_____ Occupation _____ Work Phone _____
             Postal Code

Spouse _____ Occupation _____ Work Phone _____

Name of Dentist _____ Town _____ How Long? _____

Name of Physician _____ Town _____ How Long? _____

Whom may we thank for referring you to this office? _____

Reason for visit _____

Do you have dental insurance? _____ Insurance coverage with _____

The following information is confidential and for our records only

Please check Yes or No   **Yes**   **No**

1. Are you in good health? .... ☐   ☐
2. Have you been under the care of a physician during the past 2 years? .... ☐   ☐
   Condition being treated _____
3. Date of last physical examination _____
4. Have you had any serious illness or operation? .... ☐   ☐
   If yes, what _____
5. Have you been hospitalized within the past 5 years? .... ☐   ☐
   If yes, what for _____
6. Do you have or have you had any of the following?:
   a) Rheumatic fever or rheumatic heart disease .... ☐   ☐
   b) Congenital heart lesions .... ☐   ☐
   c) Cardiovascular disease (heart trouble, heart attack, coronary insufficiency, coronary occlusion, high blood pressure, arteriosclerosis, stroke) .... ☐   ☐
      i) Do you have pain in chest upon exertion? .... ☐   ☐
      ii) Are you ever short of breath after mild exercise? .... ☐   ☐
      iii) Do your ankles swell? .... ☐   ☐
      iv) Do you get short of breath when you lie down, or do you require extra pillows when you sleep? .... ☐   ☐

	Yes	No

    v) Do you have a cardiac pacemaker? ☐ ☐

d) Allergy ☐ ☐

e) Sinus trouble ☐ ☐

f) Asthma or hay fever ☐ ☐

g) Hives or skin rash ☐ ☐

h) Fainting spells or seizures ☐ ☐

i) Diabetes ☐ ☐

    i) Do you have to urinate (pass water) more than six times a day? ☐ ☐

    ii) Are you thirsty much of the time? ☐ ☐

    iii) Does your mouth frequently become dry? ☐ ☐

j) Hepatitis, jaundice or liver disease ☐ ☐

k) Arthritis ☐ ☐

l) Inflammatory rheumatism (painful swollen joints) ☐ ☐

m) Stomach ulcers ☐ ☐

n) Kidney trouble ☐ ☐

o) Tuberculosis ☐ ☐

p) Do you have a persistent cough or cough up blood ☐ ☐

q) Low blood pressure ☐ ☐

r) Venereal disease ☐ ☐

s) Herpes infection ☐ ☐

t) Psychiatric treatment ☐ ☐

u) Epilepsy ☐ ☐

v) Hernia or eye muscle defects ☐ ☐

w) Positive testing for AIDS virus ☐ ☐

x) Contact with any situation which might increase your risk of AIDS ☐ ☐

7. Have you had abnormal bleeding associated with previous extractions, surgery, or trauma? ☐ ☐

    a) Do you bruise easily? ☐ ☐

    b) Have you ever required a blood transfusion? ☐ ☐

    If so, explain the circumstances

8. Do you have any blood disorder such as anemia? ☐ ☐

9. Have you had surgery or x-ray treatment for a tumor, growth, or other condition of your head or neck? ☐ ☐

10. Are you taking any drug or medicine? ☐ ☐

    If so, what _____

11. Are you taking any of the following?:

    a) Antibiotics or sulfa drugs ☐ ☐

    b) Anticoagulants (blood thinners) ☐ ☐

    c) Medicine for high blood pressure ☐ ☐

    d) Cortisone (steroids) ☐ ☐

    e) Tranquilizers ☐ ☐

    f) Antihistamines ☐ ☐

    g) Aspirin ☐ ☐

    h) Insulin, tolbutamide (Orinase) or similar drug ☐ ☐

    i) Digitalis or drugs for heart trouble ☐ ☐

    j) Nitroglycerin ☐ ☐

    k) Oral contraceptive or other hormonal therapy ☐ ☐

    l) Other _____ ☐ ☐

		Yes	No
12.	Are you allergic or have you reacted adversely to:		
	a) Local anesthetics	☐	☐
	b) Penicillin or other antibiotics	☐	☐
	c) Sulfa drugs	☐	☐
	d) Barbiturates, sedatives, or sleeping pills	☐	☐
	e) Aspirin	☐	☐
	f) Iodine	☐	☐
	g) Codeine or other narcotics	☐	☐
	h) Other _____		
13.	Have you had any serious trouble associated with any previous dental treatment?	☐	☐
	If so, explain _____		
	_____		
14.	Do you have any disease, condition, or problem not listed above that you think I should know about?	☐	☐
	If so, explain _____		
	_____		
15.	Are you employed in any situation which exposes you regularly to x-rays or other ionizing radiation?	☐	☐
16.	Are you wearing contact lenses?	☐	☐
17.	Have you ever had joint replacement surgery?	☐	☐
18.	Do you smoke? If so, how much _____	☐	☐

WOMEN

		Yes	No
19.	Are you pregnant?	☐	☐
20.	Do you have any problems associated with your menstrual period?	☐	☐

I understand that it is my responsibility to inform this office of any changes in my medical status.

_____   _____
Date   Signature

_____   _____
Date   Signature

SHORT MEDICAL HISTORY

Title

Name

Address

Phone numbers

Occupation

Details

1. Do you feel generally healthy? yes/no _____
2. Have you had rheumatic fever? yes/no _____
3. Have you had hepatitis or jaundice? yes/no _____
4. Do you have any heart problems such as heart attack, high blood pressure, angina, heart murmur or replacement valve? yes/no _____
5. Do you have bronchitis, asthma or other chest problems? yes/no _____
6. Are you receiving any tablets, creams, ointments from your doctor? yes/no _____
7. Have you taken any steroids in the past 2 years? yes/no _____
8. Are you allergic to any medicines, foods or other items? yes/no _____
9. Do you have arthritis? yes/no _____
10. Are you epileptic or prone to fainting? yes/no _____
11. Do you bleed excessively after cuts, extractions or other surgery? yes/no _____
12. Have you ever been hospitalized? yes/no _____
13. Have you been rejected as a blood donor? yes/no _____
14. Do you have any other medical condition we should know about? yes/no _____

Doctor's name, address and phone number

....

....

....

....

I certify that the information given is correct

Signed _____ Relationship to patient _____

MEDICO-LEGAL RELEASE FORM

I _____ (Patient's full name)

Date of Birth _____

Of _____ (Address)

_____

_____

Consent to the release of copies of my complete medical/dental records, including radiographs for the period

_____ (Dates)

to _____ (Person to be
released to)

of _____ (Address)

_____

_____

My reasons for requesting release are (this does not have to be disclosed):

_____

_____

I understand that there may be a charge for this service; I undertake that I will pay that charge

Signed _____ (Patient / Parent / Guardian /
Legal Authority)

Date _____

MEDICO-LEGAL RELEASE FORM

I _____ (Patient's full name)

Date of Birth _____

Of _____ (Address)

_____

_____

Request the release of all relevant information regarding my medical and dental health including pertinent medical/dental history, previous medical/dental treatment etc.

to _____ (Person to be released to)

of _____ (Address)

_____

_____

Signed _____ (Patient / Parent / Guardian / Legal Authority)

Date _____

MEDICO-LEGAL RELEASE FORM

Under the Terms of the Data Protection Act 1998

I _____ (Patient's full name)

Date of Birth _____

Of _____ (Address)

_____

_____

Request an appointment, under the terms of the Act within forty days, to come to the surgery to view my complete medical/dental records, including radiographs and all other data that you hold on me for the period

_____ (Dates)

Under the terms of the Act you should arrange for someone to be available to explain to me anything within those records that I do not understand

Signed _____ (Patient / Parent / Guardian /
Legal Authority)

Date _____

MEDICO-LEGAL RELEASE FORM

Under the Terms of the Data Protection Act 1998

I _____ (Patient's full name)

Date of Birth _____

Of _____ (Address)

_____

_____

Request the release of copies of my complete medical/dental records, including radiographs and all other data that you hold on me for the period

_____ (Dates)

(Under the terms of the Act this information must be released within forty days)

to _____ (Person to be released to)

of _____ (Address)

_____

_____

I understand that under the terms of the Act there will be a charge for this service; I undertake that I will pay that charge

Signed _____ (Patient / Parent / Guardian / Legal Authority)

Date _____

Index